Also from Westphalia Press
westphaliapress.org

Studies in Ethics for Nurses

by Charlotte A. Aikens

WESTPHALIA PRESS
An Imprint of Policy Studies Organization

Studies in Ethics for Nurses

Westphalia Press
An imprint of Policy Studies Organization
1527 New Hampshire Ave. NW
Washington, D.C. 20036
info@ipsonet.org

ISBN-13: 978-1-941755-10-5

Cover design by Jeffrey Barnes:
jbarnesbook.design

Daniel Gutierrez-Sandoval, Executive Director
PSO and Westphalia Press

Updated material and comments on this edition
can be found at the Westphalia Press website:
www.westphaliapress.org

STUDIES IN ETHICS FOR NURSES

BY

CHARLOTTE A. AIKENS

Formerly Superintendent of Columbia Hospital, Pittsburg, and of the Iowa Methodist Hospital, Des Moines; formerly Director of Sibley Memorial Hospital, Washington, D. C.

PHILADELPHIA AND LONDON

W. B. SAUNDERS COMPANY

1920

Published April, 1916

Reprinted September, 1916

Reprinted March and November, 1917

Reprinted April, and August, 1918

Reprinted September, 1919

Reprinted April, 1920

PRINTED IN AMERICA

PRESS OF
W. B. SAUNDERS COMPANY
PHILADELPHIA

Keep us, O God, from pettiness; let us be large in thought, in word, in deed.

Let us be done with fault-finding, and leave off self-seeking.

May we put away all pretense and meet each other face to face—without self-pity and without prejudice.

May we never be hasty in judgment and always generous.

Let us take time for all things; make us to grow calm, serene, gentle.

Teach us to put into action our better impulses, straightforward and unafraid.

Grant that we may realize it is the little things that create differences; that in the big things of life we are at one.

And may we strive to touch and to know the great, common woman's heart of us all, and,

O Lord God, let us forget not to be kind.

—Mary Stuart.

FOREWORD

The training of a nurse includes two distinct parts—distinct, yet inseparable. First, the technical instruction and experience required in the practical care of the sick and the prevention of illness. Second, the training in conduct, in ideals of personal living. The question of personal living, the ideals of character and service which a nurse holds will greatly influence her practical work every day of her nursing career.

It is easy in the pressure of training school life to devote all one's time to the first, the technical, part of a nurse's training—to subordinate the ethical to the technical, or to allow the ethical training to be crowded out entirely. Yet no amount of devotion to technical instruction will ever compensate for failure to give the nurse proper rules and principles of guidance in the moral realm; no amount of other classes which may be held will make up to a nurse what she loses, if the culture of character is forgotten during her training.

No young woman can fail to be greatly influenced by the mental and moral atmosphere in which two or three highly impressionable years of her life are passed while in training, and by the ideals of life and conduct which are shaping during those years. The fact that pupil nurses are received at an earlier age than was the case twenty years ago, and that conditions make it impossible to make the careful selection of candidates that was possible in the earlier years of training schools, calls for more systematic and careful ethical teaching than has been customary.

The purpose of this volume is to emphasize the importance of the ethical training of nurses, and to aid teachers and students in the study of conduct and duty as it relates to nurses and nursing life.

The plan of the book calls for a combination of the recitation and discussion method of class teaching. It is the author's conviction, based on observation and experience, that ten minutes which nurses are obliged to spend quietly, out of class, in the careful weighing of ethical problems, and of the far-reaching consequences of certain matters of conduct—ten minutes of serious reflection on concrete problems in which ethical principles are involved, will accomplish more in impressing them with the importance of right decisions than hours of lectures on the abstract virtues—lectures in which the nurse is simply a passive agent who is expected to absorb a certain amount of the ethical instruction she is listening to. What is most needed is that the nurse, while in training, should be obliged to *meditate* on the ethical questions likely to confront a nurse, to have those questions interpreted to her, and the lessons applied to her own life experiences. The lecture method of teaching has been tried, intermittently, for years, with exceedingly unsatisfactory results to teacher, to pupil, and to the school. Lectures have been largely abandoned in other classes in the best schools, and lectures cannot too soon be abandoned in the teaching of ethics, if results worth while are to be expected.

The requiring at intervals of written personal opinions on the methods which should be pursued in certain situations in which nurses are obliged to decide ethical questions is a valuable method in the teaching of ethics. Nurses should be trained to think things through to a logical conclusion and to be able to give reasons why they reached the decisions at which they arrived.

The teaching of ethics should begin when the pupil

enters the school, and should be carried through at regular intervals till the completion of the training period. It cannot be effectively handled by assigning a certain number of classes to it at the beginning of the training, and forgetting all about it, till the pupil is about to graduate.

For the sake of emphasis, repetition of important points has been made here and there throughout the book. There are many ethical truths which cannot be effectively taught by once telling.

The illustrations and practical problems used in the book are drawn from life, and each teacher can add to them or substitute from her own experience. The author makes no apology for revealing certain ethical failures, believing that only by the frank recognition of existing weaknesses can the weak points be strengthened; only by bringing the results of ethical failures into an open forum for discussion can conditions be improved. The only way by which the common ethical failures complained of today in nurses can ever be corrected, is by instilling in the heart of every nurse a desire to be true to her own best self; by giving each individual nurse higher standards of life and conduct, and showing her how she may reach those standards.

The author is under obligation to numerous friends in the United States and Canada who have contributed helpful suggestions from their own experience. Valuable hints have been gleaned from nursing magazines from a half dozen different countries. Three friends in the hospital and training school field have been kind enough to give critical reading to the manuscript. To name a few of these numerous friends, without naming all who have helped, would be to fail in expressing the deep appreciation felt for the counsel and very great assistance received from many different sources.

During the preparation of the volume the text-books, Principles of Ethics, by Bowne, and Social Law of Service, by Ely, have been studied. Other books referred to have been "Constructive Ethics, by Courtney; Outlines of Ethics, by Dewey; The Ethics of Personal Life, by Griggs; and Nursing Ethics, by Robb.

The author makes no claim to the production of a comprehensive treatise on the subject of Ethics for Nurses, and is fully conscious that the book has many defects. If it serves to call attention to the need of more careful ethical teaching, and more careful study by nurses of the ethical principles which should govern a life, if it helps in any measure toward bringing the ethical training and practice of nurses nearer to the ideals of life and conduct which Florence Nightingale has given to the world, it will have accomplished its mission.

CHARLOTTE A. AIKENS.

DETROIT, MICHIGAN.

CONTENTS

SECTION I

SECTION II

SECTION III

Studies in Ethics for Nurses

SECTION I

CHAPTER I

The Nurse in Her New Environment

The young woman who enters a training school for nurses finds, before proceeding far, that training in the science and art of nursing is inseparably bound up with the science and practice of moral conduct. She finds that the one phase of training influences the other at every step of the way. To attempt to teach nursing without reference to the general conduct of the individuals concerned, is like building a costly structure on a foundation of sand. Lacking a solid foundation, the structure falls when a critical moment arrives. The chief element in the foundation required to make a good nurse is to be looked for in her character. A good nurse is first of all a good woman. No amount of ability which a nurse may display in other directions can possibly be accepted as a substitute for right conduct. There is no such substitute. Taking reasonable health and intelligence for granted, the most important thing for a nurse to bring with her to the training school is a good conscience.

Foundation Principles.—The entrance of a young woman into a hospital school is, practically, the entrance into a new world—a world having laws and customs differing widely in many respects from those of the world outside, yet which are based on the same fundamental principles which govern Christian society as a whole. These principles assume the existence in every individual of a human ideal, more or less clearly perceived, and the consciousness of an obligation to maintain right and just standards of moral conduct. Ideals and standards must change and grow as civilization advances and knowledge is increased, but the foundation principles do not change. These are based on the world-old law of good will, of love to one's neighbor, of the duty to promote the general welfare of all concerned. The entrance of the nurse candidate into this new world is a rather bewildering experience, and the process of adjusting herself to these new conditions, laws, and customs is rarely easy. It may be true that duties never conflict—it is also true that to decide between apparent duties and choose the real duty for each hour and each moment, is often most confusing.

Guiding Hints.—1. An important duty for the nurse at this stage in her career is to meekly accept, as right and necessary, much that she cannot understand. 2. A second duty is to try to see every situation from the viewpoint of those in authority who have the responsibility for, and the good of the whole institution in view; also, where a patient is concerned, it is necessary to endeavor to put oneself in his place. 3. A third duty is to analyze her own motives and be sure that they are pure and unselfish, that in all things and at all times she means to do the right, as right has been revealed to her. This duty is hers, not only at the beginning of her nursing career, but all through life. The hospital must have nurses who earnestly want to do right, and who will do right as far as they see and know that a thing is right. Acoount will be taken of human frailties, allowances made for mistakes in understanding or poor judgment, but an institution for the care of the sick is no place for a girl who does not seriously want to do right—whose purpose is not fixed to do right, as far as human judgment can determine what is right under given circumstances. 4. A fourth duty, which it is important to remember at this time, is to pay careful attention to what is said by those placed in authority over the school. The careful observance of this rule will help a nurse tremendously in adjusting herself comfortably to new conditions, and in measuring up to the just expectations of those responsible for the welfare of the institution and all concerned in it.

CONCERNING GOVERNMENT

The new world which she has entered has a governing body, which is responsible to the public and to those who contribute to the support of the institution, for its proper management. This governing body may be called the board of trustees, board of managers, board of governors, or some other term, but it is the highest authority, the final court of appeal in all important matters connected with the hospital. This governing body is itself bound by certain laws and rules, designed to protect all interests concerned and to promote the general well-being of all having dealings with the institution. While, apparently, this governing body is little in evidence in the daily routine (being non-resident), it is responsible for the proper care of every patient who may be admitted, for fair and just treatment of all employed by the institution, for carrying out the purposes of the founders of the hospital, and for the wise expenditure of all money entrusted to the institution.

If a nurse makes a blunder in caring for a patient and the patient is injured or wishes to appeal to a court of law for redress, the board of managers must bear the brunt of the defense, inasmuch as they or their representatives took the responsibility of admitting the nurse to the hospital training school. They may never have seen either the nurse or the patient concerned, but they carry the responsibility for the nurse's mistakes while she is in training.

If a saucy or flippant or discourteous reply is given by a nurse to a visitor, it may seem a small thing, yet it may prove a serious disadvantage to the board in its remote effects. Large gifts have been lost to hospitals because of the carelessness or discourtesy of nurses or employees, or because of their distorted stories relative to matters which they did not fully understand. Large gifts have often come to hospitals because of the courtesy and kindness of the nursing staff.

The superintendent is the executive head of the hospital, the official representative of the board of managers in the institution, and in everyday dealings with the public. The rules and regulations pertaining to the general management and internal administration are usually arranged by him (or her) in conjunction with a committee appointed by the board for that purpose.

While he (or she) may appear to have much freedom and authority, the superintendent is nevertheless subject to limitations and rules, just as is every other member of the hospital family. He exercises only such authority as is delegated to him by the governing body.

Departments and Department Heads.—In all hospitals the work of the institutions is divided into departments, the number of departments depending somewhat on the size of the place, and the character of the work done.

The administration department is the center of the system. It may be compared to the hub of the wheel, with the various departments representing the spokes. The superintendent is the official head of the administration department. The assistant superintendent assumes such duties as are assigned by the superintendent.

The departments found in most hospitals are:

1. *The medical department* composed of the medical staff, visiting physicians, internes, and other medical assistants. It has to do with the medical and surgical care of patients.

2. *The nursing department* or the training school, under which are grouped all nurses actively engaged in nursing, all probationers, the orderlies, and all other employees who are assisting in the work of this department. This department is usually the largest in point of numbers.

3. *The domestic or housekeeping department* deals with matters relating to the housing of the hospital household, the cleaning and general care of the building, and the laundry. In most hospitals the feeding of the hospital family and of those connected with this work also comes under this department. In larger institutions this may be a separate department having its own separate head and staff of workers, and is known as the dietary department.

4. *The engineer's department* has to do with heating, lighting, and ventilation of the building, and with other related matters. Not all hospitals have their duties and responsibilities divided in the same manner.

5. *Other Departments.*—The out-patient department usually includes the social service department. The pathological department and the drug department are other departments commonly found in larger hospitals.

In smaller hospitals the superintendent is often obliged

to assume responsibilities which in larger hospitals are divided among several people.

While each of these departments has its own head, the administration department has to do with all departments. There is no part of the building or grounds which should not be under the watchful eye of the superintendent; no part in which he (or she) is not and should not be actively interested; no department in which he is not entirely justified in making suggestions or giving directions in regard to its management. He (or she) usually is superintendent of the whole institution, and is expected by the board of governors to oversee every part of it. His requests should have all the force of commands.

Service.—All these departments working together spell S E R V I C E in a very real and vital meaning of the term. Service to our fellow-beings is the object of the institution. It is expected to be the object of every individual connected with it. If a nurse does not bring with her, when she enters the school, the spirit of helpful service, she has made a mistake in the step she has taken. She should choose some other occupation.

The patient is the most important person in the entire institution. He is the reason for its existence. His welfare and his comfort are and should always be given first consideration. Without patients there is no need of these various departments, and, throughout a nurse's whole career, the patient's welfare while she is in charge should never be placed in the background of her thought or plans.

While the new world which the probationer has entered may seem to be made up of a miscellaneous collection of people—engineers, firemen, laundresses, ambulance men, porters, ward maids, cooks, head nurses, doctors, internes, druggists, bookkeepers, clerks, etc.—each one fits into his own department, is subject to the rules of that department, and is expected to do his part faithfully and well in the institutional plans. The carelessness or blunder of one member of these varied groups may easily upset the smooth running of the whole human machinery of the institution.

For example, the failure of the kitchen workers to have breakfast ready on time may easily upset the smooth working of the whole institution. Failure in the laundry is quickly felt in the wards and operating rooms. Failure of nurses to attend to the sending back of soiled dishes at the proper time throws the plans of kitchen workers into confusion. Thus illustrations might be multiplied to show how dependent one department is on another, and how necessary it is for all to work harmoniously together.

This explains the reason for the various rules and regulations which every hospital is obliged to enforce in order that negligence in one department shall not hinder the work of other departments. Not all the human units are equally important, but unless each person is of some importance, there is no reason for his being a part of the service.

Individual Responsibility.—In this new world of the hospital, individuals are valued, largely, according to their ability to carry responsibility. This feeling of responsibility for faithful doing of her own tasks and also for faithfulness to the larger interests of the institution is something which a nurse should try to cultivate from her first probation day. It has more to do with her full and final success than she can possibly realize at the beginning of her career. The nurse who feels keenly her personal responsibility is the nurse who is trusted and depended on, and who, later, has larger responsibilities committed to her.

The Spirit of the Training School.—It was previously stated that the patient was the most important part of the institution. He is also the reason for the existence of most of the rules and customs which have come into existence in hospitals. Most of these rules and customs are designed directly or indirectly to promote the patient's welfare and to guide those who have the responsibility for his care. For example, the rule requiring nurses to be in bed at a proper hour at night is designed primarily to safeguard the nurse's own health, but in spirit it extends to the welfare of the patients, because it is well known that a nurse who has not had sufficient rest and sleep lowers her efficiency as a nurse, is more liable to mistakes, and the welfare of the patient suffers. Thus, when rule after rule is analyzed, each will be found, in most cases, to have its root in the safety and comfort of patients and the well-being of all concerned.

Concerning Loyalty.—Loyalty to the institution on the part of nurses, employees, and all who form a part of its working staff, is one of its most valuable assets. It is also one of the most important essentials to the efficient service which the hospital owes to the public whom it serves. It is one of the working principles of all such institutions that acceptance of contracts for service, or to enter the institution as a student or in any other capacity, carries with it the spoken or unspoken pledge of loyalty to the institution. Whether the period of one's connection with the hospital be long or short, it is better both for the hospital and for the workers themselves that all whose duty it is to interpret the spirit of the hospital to the public should be loyal rather than disloyal.

Loyalty does not mean that one must shut one's eyes to the shortcomings of the institution. No institution is perfect. Its work has to be done by very human individuals who are far from perfect. It does mean that one who is loyal will refrain from fault-finding or criticism except where criticism is made to those who are in a position to remedy it. It means that a nurse will not mention the failings or defects of her associates to the patients or to outside people. It means, where a patient or some one from outside the institution complains, that the loyal member of the hospital household will defend the interests of the institution just as she would defend the interests of her own home. It is highly desirable for the good of the patient that his confidence in the hospital should not be shaken. Loyalty to the institution involves much more than this. It means that one who is loyal to an institution will be careful to observe its rules; that the property of the hospital will not be misused; that its officers will be treated with respect; that courtesy will be rendered to all; and that each worker will remember that she has the reputation and welfare of the hospital to a certain extent in her keeping.

Loyalty to the physician is one of the duties demanded of every nurse, not solely because the physician is her superior officer, but chiefly because the confidence of the patient in his physician is one of the important elements in the management of his illness, and nothing should be said or done that would weaken this faith or create doubts as to the character or ability or methods of the physician on whom he is depending.

Loyalty to the patient's welfare demands, first of all, that his rights be respected and that his private affairs shall not be discussed with other patients or with people outside the hospital. This includes refraining from discussing patients or hospital matters with outside nurses, with close friends, with members of one's own family, or with any other individuals with whom a nurse associates, except those professionally concerned.

The Hospital Atmosphere.—In all institutions there is present that subtle intangible thing called atmosphere, and the nurse, in common with all others, is affected by it, though often unconscious that she is being affected. The spirit or tone of the institution depends much on those in authority. It depends somewhat on the primary aims of the place. It depends greatly on the workers, the spirit which they put into their tasks, and their general mental attitude toward the work they have undertaken.

While the nurse is passing through the wards or attending classes, she is catching the influence of the personalities with whom she is associated, but she is not a passive individual. From the time she enters the hospital, she herself is impressing *her* ideals and standards on others and is helping to create the moral atmosphere in which she and others move. The hospital will be made better or worse by her presence in it, by the way she does her work, by her daily conduct, on and off duty, by what she says, and by her general moral and spiritual influence. What she is counts for more than what she does.

The spirit of the nurse as she reveals it, unconsciously, day by day in the wards, in the corridors, in her room, in the class room, at meals, and in off-duty times, is another of the important points in which she will be judged during her probation, and later by the public, as she takes her place in the busy world outside. It manifests itself in a thousand different ways. Some one has said that one of the first and hardest lessons a nurse has to learn is to spell SELF with a little s.

It is often difficult for her to realize that success and advancement in this work, as in many others, usually comes to the one who continually studies how he may give his fellow-beings a little more, a little better, service.

Suggestions for Written Work.—In a paper of between 200 and 300 words give an outline of your life since your fourteenth year, mentioning the responsibilities you have had, and your reasons for desiring a nurse's training. Have papers ready for class to be held—

FOR DISCUSSION OR REVIEW

1. Mention two fundamental principles that should govern in civilized and Christian society.
2. What is an ideal? Of what value is it in life?
3. State four guiding hints given in the preceding chapter to help a nurse in adjusting herself to the new world of the training school.
4. In your estimation which of these guiding hints should be placed first in its importance to be observed during probation? Give reasons for your answer.
5. State some of the important responsibilities which the governing board of a hospital carry.
6. Mention several ways by which a nurse may seriously embarrass the governing body.
7. By what term is the official head of the hospital usually known? Tell what you know of his relation to the various departments.
8. For what do the various departments of the hospital exist?
9. Whom do you consider the most important person in the hospital? Why?
10. Mention one special quality in a nurse which largely determines her value as a worker.

11. Show why it is necessary for the welfare of the patient that he have confidence in the institution and in those who are responsible for his care.

12. What do you understand by the phrase "loyalty to an institution?"

13. State, briefly, several ways in which the spirit which a nurse manifests in everyday life may influence her success as a nurse.

14. How may a nurse help in securing or maintaining the right moral atmosphere in a hospital?

CHAPTER II

The Nurse Herself

Since the nurse is the person to be trained, and since she herself will have a large part in the training of her own powers, it is very necessary that she make a careful study of herself, her possibilities, her ambitions, her general make-up. She needs to know of some of the difficulties she is likely to encounter in the process of making an acceptable nurse out of very human material, which is such a mixture of good and bad, of strength and weakness, of high and low impulses, striving for the mastery in the human heart. A nurse is successful and effective in her work not only by what she knows how to do, but by what she is. Call this study psychology, if you will, but do not neglect it.

Few young women realize that learning how to perform nursing duties is the smallest part of the training process, that the drilling and disciplining of the woman inside the nurse, the development of right character, a right attitude of mind, and habits of life, is the most difficult part in the making of a nurse.

Personality, that intangible thing that distinguishes us from every other individual, exercises a powerful influence over the sick for whom we care, and also over the well people with whom we associate. Nature has endowed each of us with certain gifts and qualities and tendencies. The development of those gifts and qualities which are good, the checking or correcting of tendencies that are detrimental, the strengthening of our weak points, the cultivation of a pleasing personality, or the reverse, depends more on the nurse herself than on any one else.

It is easy for a nurse to degenerate morally and spiritually while in training in spite of all the moral safeguards the school affords. In the important transition period of her life through which she is passing she needs to "hold fast to that which is good" and to watch that she does not retrograde, that she does not lose out of her heart life the things which no woman can afford to lose who desires to be "a good woman" in the highest, deepest, broadest and best sense of the term.

The Will.—The nurse's will, the faculty or endowment of the soul by which it is capable of making a choice, the power of the mind by which she decides to do or not to do, is the great test of character and life. The training of the will until right habits are formed, and certain courses are taken, or things done unconsciously or without effort of will, is at the bottom of character building. Its results are shown in what a nurse does, not in what she thinks or intends.

Inclination is sometimes confused with the will, but it is a less significant term, meaning simply a disposition more favorable to one thing than another. We may easily be inclined to do a thing, yet fail to do it. A nurse makes her record in a hospital by what she does, not by what she is inclined to do.

Ambition.—An eager desire for the attainment of certain objects is an important element in the making of a nurse, yet it may easily become an inordinate desire for preferment, honor, position, or power of some kind. Ambition is a quality which every individual should cultivate, yet diligently keep under control. It should help to carry a nurse forward to greater achievements, yet not at the expense of others. The finest ambition is that which leads a nurse to overcome obstacles and difficulties, rather than to outreach competitors. The man or woman who wins is often the one who revels in working at, or working out, hard things which others are ready to give up.

It is easy to be *an average nurse;* it costs to be the finest kind, in character, life and general attainments, along any line we may choose.

One of the most wonderful pianists in America, one whose technic is marvelous, whose soul is full of harmonies, was asked how he came to be such a musician. "I gave myself up to music," he replied. "For three years I sat before my piano from morning until night. I rarely went anywhere. I saw almost no friends. I lived for my music. I know I lost much in a social way, but I wanted above everything else to be a master musician." And he is. But it cost. It meant giving up lesser things for something which he greatly desired.

It is neither wise nor necessary for nurses to cut themselves off from all social life; they need it, they need friends—friends and acquaintances who are not of the world of sickness in which they live—but it is well to remember that it costs to be a high-grade nurse in character and habits and attainments. The nurse who is unwilling to study or sacrifice, who comes to the hospital "to see if she will like it," who feels that social pleasures or her engagements should take precedence to duty, needs either to change her attitude of mind or to choose some other line of work that will leave her free to make social engagements and do as she pleases with her time. She does not desire to be a nurse strongly enough to pay the price cheerfully. The readiness or reluctance with which a sacrifice of personal feeling is made is a revelation of character which those who are training nurses are quick to observe in probationers. Think why this is so.

Temper.—Early in the training course the nurse learns that she must never argue with a patient; that she must learn to get along sweetly with others; that she must learn to control her temper. She knows or should know that the nurse who flies off in anger at trifles must acquire self-control, must master her feelings, or she will always be under a handicap as a nurse or as a worker in any line of activity. Anger is usually looked on as a serious evil in life, yet anger has its place. The man or woman who can't get angry when occasion arises, who can't feel deeply indignant, is made of poor material. Yet it needs no argument to convince us that anger indulged in frequently or habitually is a sign of personal weakness, a sign that the individual has not learned to rule his own spirit, that he who indulges in anger hurts himself.

Is it easier for some nurses to be sweet-tempered than others? Watch those with whom you associate and decide for yourself. What is the chief secret of a sweet sunny temper? How may it be cultivated? Think it over and try to give a satisfactory answer to yourself.

Quite as disturbing sometimes as anger are the signs of irritability or impatience one sometimes sees in nurses. The well-controlled nurse will not often give way to outbursts of impatience. The provocation many times will be great, yet the temptation to give vent to one's feeling in a snappy answer must be held in check. What would be the general atmosphere in a hospital if everyone followed the example of the nurse who, when busy with a bed patient, was asked by a patient in an adjoining bed to give her a glass of water? Without stopping to think how it sounded or what the effect on the patient or the ward would be the nurse snapped out: "Can't you see I'm busy? I haven't got three hands." This sort of temptation nurses will have to meet every day, and the way in which they meet these everyday tests will show whether or not they have in them good nursing material.

Habit.—When an act has been repeated so frequently that it is done almost spontaneously without much previous thought, it is spoken of as a habit. Scientists have stated that the current of thought moving in the same direction for a time has worn a groove in the plastic brain material, and that this groove is deepened as the act is repeated until it becomes almost automatic for the thought to take that course. It requires no conscious effort.

Even superficial consideration of the matter will show how much of our lives is made up of habit, and how important it is to cultivate right habits in nursing and personal life. No course of action is trifling if it has in it the possibility of habit formation.

We are influenced, partly unconsciously, to the formation of habits by the example and influence of those with whom we live in daily contact, and especially by the example of those in authority. Our attitude of mind is influenced by their attitude, but our wills are given to us to help keep us from forming wrong habits of body or of mind. We may love people without copying their faults.

While these lines are being penned there lies before the writer a remarkable copy of a journal edited by the prisoners in one of the state penitentiaries.* It has a

* From Joliet Prison Post.

department known as "The Guide Post," over which appears this inscription: "One turn to the Right, then Straight On." The editor of the Guide Post department states the following truths which, perhaps, sound strangely coming from a man confined in a state's prison, but they are some of the great truths of life which all need to remember. He says: "There is a word in the English language which has a peculiar power. It is Righteousness, and it seems to be at the very bottom of all things. Should it seem pleasing not to do so, it is not necessary to associate this word with any creed, orthodoxy or dogma. It is simply something thorough. But to find it, one must let truth illuminate the road.

"Conscience is to the soul what health is to the body. No man knows what conscience is until he understands what solitude can teach him about it.

"As to the future, let us cast new resolutions to the winds; they are too often shallow and meaningless. But let us hearken to that inner voice that requireth every man to mean well and to do his best in the world.

"Let us cultivate those traits and habits which make for character, for character is the governing element of life. It cannot be constructed; it needs first of all a principle and an impulse, glowing and determined."

Think carefully over the quotations from the prisoner's journal. Underline the sentences or phrases which you deem most important. Ask yourself why they seem important to you. Do you agree with the prisoner's philosophy at every point?

Suggestions for Written Work.—Prepare a short paper describing what you think is a proper ideal of character for a nurse to keep before her during her first year of training, and what she should do in order to reach her ideal.

FOR DISCUSSION OR REVIEW

1. Show why you believe that a nurse has a large part in the training of herself.

2. What do you mean by the term "personality?" In what way does it influence a nurse's success? Has a nurse any control over her personality?

3. What is the difference between "will" and "inclination?"

4. What has ambition to do with the quality of nursing service? What dangers may there be in having too great ambition?

5. Is there such a thing as righteous anger? Give an example. What place has anger in dealing with patients?

6. What is habit? How are habits formed?

7. Mention some precautions which nurses should exercise in regard to habit.

8. What is conscience? What effect does it have on the life and work of a nurse?

CHAPTER III

Expressions of Personality

When we speak of a well-poised woman we mean one who is physically, mentally and morally well balanced; one whose best powers have been developed symmetrically in a proper way; one who avoids going to extremes, and who has an innate sense of the proportionate value of things in general.

Poise of soul comes from careful thinking, from meditation on the great principles which affect personal life and living. It manifests itself in numerous ways. It is a thing to be striven for by every nurse. The possession of poise, or the lack of it, affects tremendously the estimation in which an individual is held by the people whose respect she desires to secure. It means more than self-control. A stoic may be self-controlled, but he may be absolutely without heart. He may be able to maintain a stoical demeanor because he is indifferent, absolutely unconcerned, as to the issues involved, even though they may be tremendously important to others.

Self-control.—It is soon recognized that nurses need to cultivate the habit of not being easily excited. They quickly learn that self-control is indispensable. They should also learn that it does not necessarily mean a lack of sympathy or a callous indifferent disposition, but a mind and body brought under the control of the will and trained to express sympathy in a very practical way.

An unknown writer in a city daily, writing on the subject of self-control, says:

"Many an individual has seen fleeting opportunity elude his grasp because at the moment the self-control necessary to intelligent reaching was not his.

"Self-control means precisely what it reads—the full command of yourself, the captaincy over your mind and body under military discipline.

"It means to be able to hold yourself in check when natural inclination would overstep the bounds of common sense. It means quite as well to be able to speed yourself up when natural inclination unwisely lags. It is both brake and throttle under your hand.

"It is more. It is steering wheel, too. It is the mental poise which enables you to scan guide posts and turns in the road without too much prejudice or predilection, but rather with an open-mindedness that invites and recognizes reason.

"Self-control keeps you from fighting when peace is of greater moment, and from peace when fighting is needed. It keeps you from doing the unwise thing when emotion or lack of patience or momentary weakness or outside pressure would lead you into indiscretions of temper or speech or action.

"Self-control wins many victories, but makes few enemies. And it is a great conserver of self-respect. It never cheapens its possessor.

"Self-control—control of self.

"It's not easy. It's hard. It's harder than controlling someone else. If you're in a position to command, the others must obey. But when it comes to commanding yourself—obedience is only a matter of experiment. If you can control yourself you are doubly strong."

Analyze this quotation. Show where you agree with

the writer. How does one's early training influence the matter of self-control?

The expression of the face, the tone of voice, and the character of our touch all affect materially for good or ill the patient's comfort and condition. The patient who is anxious about his condition will study carefully the expression of the face of doctor or nurse to see if he can discern from the face what the opinion is which they do not openly express in words. Therefore control of the expression of the face and of the voice, so that neither face nor voice expresses anxiety, alarm, or surprise, however serious the occasion may be, is one of the important lessons a nurse must learn. Tone and manner often convey more than the spoken word.

A sudden exclamation of surprise may so alarm a patient as to greatly hinder his chance of fighting a winning battle at a critical time, by giving rise to fear and mental anxiety; therefore the face must be trained not to tell tales, and the exclamation of surprise must often be repressed.

It is, however, not necessary or desirable to always repress the expression of pleasure or gladness, either in face or voice, when all is going well. A happy quality of optimism in a nurse is an element much to be desired, and it can be cultivated.

The Voice.—The quality of the voice may seem to a nurse something which she cannot control, something with which she was born and for which she is not responsible, yet a little thought and study of herself will convince her that habit has much to do with it. A nurse may be habitually loud-voiced or gentle-voiced when she enters the school and may never have had attention called to it. She must train herself to realize that her habits of voice influence greatly the comfort of the patients and also their appreciation of her value as a nurse. She must discipline her voice if she does not wish, many times, to be considered a nuisance. It is hard to imagine the amount of unnecessary discomfort that the sick are obliged to suffer because of the undisciplined voice in nurses, and because of the thoughtless chatter that is so often heard in corridors. Study your own voice. Do you speak distinctly, firmly, yet gently; or do you drawl your words out as if you had no energy behind them? Is your voice, or habit of speaking, harsh, discordant or unnecessarily loud? Is your tone quick, sharp, shrill; has it that piercing quality which jars sensitive nerves and often causes real pain? Do you mumble your words or speak in whispers? Do your tones indicate a cheerful, kindly disposition or the opposite? Have your tones that quiet, gentle, firm note of authority and strength which inspires confidence? Have you ever tried to cultivate the habit of speaking gently, quietly, distinctly? When you read aloud have you ever tried to discover whether your voice was agreeable and pleasant, or discordant or monotonous, or whether it had that singsong quality which ought to be corrected? Nurses may help each other much by reminding each other of points at which they need to be especially careful.

Touch and Movement.—Instinctively we feel that a nurse should be gentle, yet habitual gentleness requires a real effort and includes much. Few defects in a nurse are more quickly noted by patients or observers than the lack of gentleness. A nervous self-conscious nurse often jars the bed and the patient, slams doors, drops things, and unnecessarily causes suffering till the strangeness of the new situation wears off. This is excusable at the beginning. It becomes a serious defect if it continues.

The size and shape of the hands are usually settled before we enter a training school. The quality of touch is under our control. By the touch we may convey to the patient our feeling of sympathy and tenderness, our appreciation of his weakened condition, our desire to be helpful. We reveal our character in our touch, to a considerable extent.

The human hand has in it a wonderful power to soothe tired nerves; its subtle influence over the mind cannot easily be explained. It can easily be used in such a way as to indicate familiarity of manner, against which a nurse needs to guard with all patients.

Three things especially to be studied in movement are: gentleness, deftness, quickness.

Carriage.—Just as the voice and touch reveal character, so the manner in which a nurse walks and carries herself will reveal the habits of the woman and will exert a very real if undefinable influence on the sick. "*Stand straight*" and "*sit straight*" are admonitions frequently needed by nurses. An erect carriage, an air of alertness, a keen attitude of attention are evidences of a well-disciplined body and of a certain general culture. These can be acquired, but not without effort.

Habits to be avoided are a careless attitude in standing, as if the backbone were weak and needed support; a lounging posture in sitting; leaning against the bed or other support; sitting on the patient's bed.

The character of the walk is a matter to be studied by every nurse. It also reveals to some extent the mental attitude of the woman. A quick, energetic nurse usually thinks and moves quickly. Others are slower in grasping ideas and usually slower in their walk and general movements. Women who are indolent by nature reveal it in their carriage, walk, and general movements.

Heavy, loud footsteps in a nurse are indications of a certain lack in the mental qualities desirable. Habits of walking to be avoided are the mincing gait; tip-toeing; the quick, nervous walk which is a half run and which betokens a nurse who is flurried; the dragging footstep and the heavy thud.

A quiet, even, steady, firm walk which can be quickened on occasion is the least wearing on a nurse and most satisfactory for everybody concerned. A light footfall comes naturally to some people. Needless to say every nurse should wear a comfortable broad-soled shoe with rubber heels while on duty.

The Uniform.—The uniform has been adopted as a necessary part of the nurse's equipment. It announces to the little world in which the wearer lives and works the character of her duties in the institution. It carries with it a certain quality that helps to dignify the wearer and demands a certain respect.

Does a nurse stop to consider that the manner in which she wears the uniform is an index of character? However carefully the school authorities may design a uniform, it can be worn so as to present a careless, untidy appearance. If there are pins where buttons were intended; if the skirt is bedraggled and frayed at the edges; if the nurse has so little sense of the fitness of things that she is found wearing rings or other unnecessary jewelry with a uniform dress that is designed for work; if her hair is untidy, her cap crooked, or perched in a fly-away fashion on her head, so that it attracts undue attention; if part of the uniform is always missing, may we not conclude that such a nurse is lacking in attention to details and apt to be as careless in her work as in her appearance?

A proper uniform includes more than dress, apron, cap,

collars and cuffs. It requires due attention to the amount of starch used in laundering. It should be so made as to allow freedom in movement to the wearer. It should be noiseless. There should be no cuffs with sharp edges that may be uncomfortable to the patient. Any elaborate style of hair dressing is out of place with the uniform. It calls for neatness and cleanliness from head to foot. It is limited to the details prescribed by the school. A well-trained nurse with her sense of what is proper duly developed will not be found wearing rings on fingers or in ears, bracelets, hair adornments, or conspicuous footgear, while on duty in hospital or home.

It is entirely probable that the probationer has rarely, if ever, before entering the school, taken time to really think seriously on the subject of her own personality, and the thousand ways in which she is revealing it every day. She needs now to study herself, the failings and habits and tendencies which she should try to correct, as she never did before. Only a few of the ways in which character is revealed have been mentioned. Others will be discussed later on, but let it never be forgotten that the soul of the woman who wears the uniform will influence the quality of her work, every day that she lives.

Suggested Subject for Written Work.—Prepare a short paper on the question, "What is training as it relates to nursing?" stating your ideas of what training should accomplish in you, apart from learning to give practical bodily care to the sick.

FOR DISCUSSION OR REVIEW

1. When you speak of a well-poised woman, what do you mean?
2. How may poise of soul be cultivated?

3. Show how poise may differ from self-control.

4. In the practice of self-control, mention some things to be guarded against.

5. State why you believe that self-control is indispensable to a nurse.

6. Mention several ways in which the expression of a nurse's face may affect the mental attitude of the patient.

7. How may a nurse's voice affect the comfort of patients?

8. What qualities of voice should a nurse cultivate? What qualities avoid?

9. Show how touch, movement and manner of walking may reveal character.

10. Mention three qualities of movement which nurses should try especially to cultivate.

11. Why do nurses wear uniforms? Mention some things that should be avoided in the wearing of the uniform.

12. Give some reasons why rings and other jewelry are out of place on a nurse in uniform.

CHAPTER IV

Conduct and Duty

One of the main purposes of this text-book is *to make nurses think*, think hard and frequently, about questions of conduct and duty. In the long career, the nurse's ideals of conduct and of duty are the biggest factors in her success, professionally and financially. It cannot be too deeply impressed on a nurse that her own ambitions and ideals, the spirit which she puts into her work, will be the chief determining factors in fixing her status in the great working world.

Analyzing an Ideal.—It is well, then, at the beginning that a nurse should have a fairly clear idea of the kind of nurse she wishes to become. Her ideals will grow and change with the passing years, but, since she herself has a most important part in the training process, it is very desirable that she try to have a clear conception of the kind of nurse she is anxious to be. Let her think of the nurses she has known and read of, study the characteristics she admires in each, and also the characteristics which she thinks should be avoided. It is much better for the nurse to take a real person and try to analyze her habits and spirit than to frame a theoretical ideal which might not fit any woman who ever lived, on earth or in heaven.

What do you know of the illustrious founder of modern nursing, Florence Nightingale, of the qualities that made her great? What did she do in order to fit herself to improve nursing conditions? What difficulties did she encounter? What sort of woman was she, as a woman, apart from her nursing? What do you most admire in her character? What nurses have you met whom you admired greatly, whom you wished to be like, and what was it that you admired? What qualities have you seen expressed in a nurse's life or conduct that you feel should be avoided or corrected?

It is easy for any of us to sit down and write out a description of an abstract ideal for a nurse, but what we want are examples of real nurses, living or dead, who had to meet the everyday difficulties the nurse of today meets and yet made their lives in aims and habits safe examples to follow.

Ethics Defined.—The nurse in her probation period and all through her career will hear much about "ethics;" therefore it is well at the outset that she try to understand what is included in the term. Dictionaries define ethics as the science which deals with moral conduct or with human duty. The meaning of the word covers custom, usage, habits, and in its application commonly refers to personal characteristics, or to the traditions of a community. As related to nursing, ethics has to do with the ideals, customs and habits which the members of the profession are by degrees accumulating around the name and character of the trained nurse.

Nursing Habits.—The importance of correcting bad habits and forming good ones was mentioned in a preceding chapter. While we speak and think of nursing habits as usually formed during training, it is a fact that the habits which we form during training are largely dependent on the habits we brought with us to the training school, the habits which were forming during childhood, and which had become more or less fixed before coming to the training school. What are some of those habits? Are you energetic, alert, or inclined to be lazy and careless? Are you neat and gentle, or untidy and inclined to be noisy? Are you, as a rule, punctual in getting to church on time and in keeping appointments, or do you dawdle and act as if punctuality was of no special importance and you didn't care whose time you wasted by being late? These are examples of some of the habits which a nurse brings with her to the training school.

What is sympathy? How much place has in it a nurse's life? Should it be repressed or cultivated? What sort of a heart and head should a nurse try to bring with her to the school?

When you speak of an obliging disposition, just what do you mean? To what extent is a nurse responsible for the disposition she manifests?

What is included in the term "a pleasing personality," and how much does "a pleasing personality" have to do with nursing? Do you consider respect for authority a desirable quality for a nurse to cultivate? If so, why?

Helps toward Right Habits.—In beginning the new life in the hospital, it is very necessary and desirable to cling to all the helps we can possibly get, which may aid in the formation of right habits. It has been stated that the thousands of new laws passed by state legislatures every year are all based to a degree on the ten commandments and the great commandment—"Thou shalt love the Lord thy God with all thy heart and with all thy soul and with all thy strength and with all thy mind, and thy neighbor as thyself." Since the Bible has given to most of us, either directly or indirectly, the highest and best laws and rules of life and conduct, it is very necessary that when we enter the training school we bring our Bibles, or other devotional books with us, and that we do not allow any other study, or any number of them, to crowd the best things out of our lives. This is one mistake which nurses frequently make. There has probably never been a time in their lives when they needed, quite so much, the helps which religion affords, as when they are in the training period and in the transition state, when new temptations, new problems of duty confront them on every side; and never a time in their lives when it will seem easier to grow careless about securing spiritual help, and find a reasonably good excuse for so doing.

Next among the helps to right conduct and right living, let us place the old-fashioned habit of going to church—the church of our home training, or to synagogue, or to services, where we will get for ourselves the uplifting influences of public worship. Every nurse needs this to keep her from growing hard and callous, to help her to keep her mind from running always in the same channel, to help her to be sweet and sane, winning and optimistic, and to exert a wholesome influence in the little circle in which she moves.

The Roots of Ethical Teaching.—When we get close enough to study beneath the surface we will probably discover that the subject of ethics in some respects resembles a tree, with roots deep down and with branches out in several directions. If we do not notice the roots of the tree we may expect to develop branches and fruit and have them flourish without roots. The roots of the tree we may designate as Religion which some writer has said is "the relation which an individual fixes between his soul and his God." "The fruits of the spirit, love, joy, peace, long-suffering, gentleness, goodness, faith, meekness, temperance," are fruits greatly to be desired in a nurse's daily life, but it is hard for them to flourish without diligent cultivation.

Concerning Conscience.—Among the fundamental requirements for the making of a good nurse we have placed the matter of conscience. It influences her work, at every turn of the way, both in the hospital and in the great world outside. Do nurses enter the training school with equally well-developed, sensitive consciences? If a good, healthy, sensitive conscience is a necessity for a good nurse, how can she acquire it if she did not have a well-developed conscience on entrance? This seems like a thoroughly important question for a nurse to consider. Did the ideal nurse whom you analyzed at the beginning of this chapter have a good active conscience, or not?

Ethics and Health.—The subject of ethics enters into the secret places of one's life. Ethics does not concern itself simply with abstract ideals and virtues. The subject is as broad and deep as life itself. It has a very close relation to a nurse's own health, and her conception of her ethical obligations may have a very real bearing on the health of those committed to her care. Her carelessness in health matters may easily create unnecessary burdens for those who are responsible for the nursing in the hospital

The nurse who neglects the hygienic precautions which she knows should be observed may easily carry infection from one patient to another, may add to the burden of sickness which they are already carrying, and may endanger life itself. There is a very real relation between a nurse's conscience and infection, even though the subjects at first glance may seem wide apart.

Where Special Precautions are Needed.—Two very important parts of a nurse's anatomy which need careful guarding to keep them in good condition are her hands and her feet. From the beginning of her career in the care of the sick, she should practice the habit of avoiding touching with her hands as far as possible dressings, basins or materials of any kind that are liable to contain disease-producing germs. Under the finger nails is a favorite lurking place for germs and the careless nurse, however good her intentions may be, may easily, by being careless about her hands, carry infection into her own body as well as infect others. Careful cleansing of the hands before meals or before partaking of food of any kind is a rule that cannot be too closely observed. Soap and water applied to the hands freely and frequently are powerful safeguards to the health of a nurse. She has it in her own power to ward off much sickness. If she is careless and does not use the safeguards which are at her disposal, she must bear a considerable part of the blame when sickness overtakes her. As a rule, nurses are as happy and healthy a class of young women as are found in any school or college. Many nurses have gone through their entire course of training without missing one day on account of sickness. This is the ideal a nurse should have. Breaks in the skin of the hand, hang nails, minor cuts, etc., should be carefully attended to, as they afford an avenue for the entrance of infectious germs to the body.

Since much of a nurse's work requires standing or walking, the condition of the feet is of prime importance. Most schools require a nurse to bring with her a pair of comfortable well-fitting shoes with low heels, for ward duty. A few schools have the feet of all nurses examined and special shoes prescribed. Apart entirely from the matter of comfort, which is highly important, it is plain that no nurse is at her best, nor in condition to do her best for her patient, if she is suffering tortures from tight, badly fitting, or unsuitable shoes.

The nurse's duty to herself should never be overlooked. It is just as real as her duty to others. Neither should it be given undue prominence in our consideration. To have a proper sense of proportion, giving due importance to certain things and placing less important things where they belong in our plans, is highly necessary for effective service. In the classes in hygiene attention will be given to details which affect personal health. At the beginning it is very desirable that a nurse get a proper attitude of mind in regard to health, the relation of her health to the plans and management of the institution, and to the occupation which she has chosen. In every class of a dozen probationers there are likely to be found three types of nurses:

1. Those who give up and go to bed for very slight, and sometimes fancied ailments.

2. Those who will persistently assert that they are not ill and who remain on duty when their own common sense tells them they should be in bed.

3. Those who take a sensible middle ground and, when they do not feel as well as usual, frankly come and report the matter to those in charge, realizing that slight indisposition, if attended to promptly, may prevent suffering and loss of time to the nurse herself, and inconvenience to those who have to assume her duties if she has to be sent to bed.

No training school can afford to carry through an extended period of training a nurse who is likely to disrupt the machinery every few weeks by reporting on the sick list. It is unfair to the other nurses who must assume her duties while she is laid aside, and unfair to those who will later on employ her. There are other occupations which such women should take up, where less vital issues will depend on their uncertain health.

On the other hand, it is well for nurses to remember that principals and head nurses much prefer to know that a nurse is not feeling well, so that prompt measures may be taken to correct what is wrong, and they cannot be expected to know of such things unless they are told. Experience quickly enables them, as a rule, to see whether the indisposition is trifling and likely to pass off soon, or whether it is something needing careful attention at once. Many nurses are subject to frequent attacks of sore throat. Hospital life occasionally seems to aggravate this trouble and special precautions should be practised. Especially should they be careful to mention to the principal of the school the first symptoms of the approach of this ailment. In spite of the emphasis which is placed on this matter of telling when the first symptoms of sore throat are felt, one frequently finds a nurse who will foolishly disobey or ignore the instructions given her till she is forced to go to bed with tonsillitis, and will give as her reason that she hesitated to trouble anyone. She neglects to look far enough ahead to see that if she is obliged to go off duty and be cared for, she will be causing much more trouble than if she had obeyed the instructions she received.

Suggestions for Written Work.—A probationer was told to report for duty at the hospital on the morning of July 8. Instead, she came to the city with a friend, spent two days in sight-seeing and visiting, and reported at the hospital on the evening of July 9. What handicaps did she place on herself at the beginning of her career? What estimate would the principal of the school be likely to place on her value as a student and worker? What important principle which she should have observed did she violate at the beginning of her training?

QUESTIONS FOR DISCUSSION OR REVIEW

1. Mention two factors which affect powerfully a nurse's success, professionally and financially.

2. Describe the nurse you have met who came nearest to your ideal.

3. What do you understand by the phrase "ethics of nursing?"

4. Make a list of things which are helpful to the formation of right habits.

5. What book is the basis for most of the laws of the world and the ideals of right conduct? Explain what is meant by the Golden Rule.

6. Mention some advantages of church going as a habit.

7. What suggestions would you offer a nurse in regard to conscience building?

8. Can you trace any relation between ethics and health as it relates to nurses and nursing?

9. Outline some precautions which nurses should use in the care of their hands and their feet.

10. Show how a nurse's carelessness in matters of health may disrupt the plans of the nursing department.

CHAPTER V

Old-fashioned Virtues

The nurse who enters a hospital for training comes, or should come, with a conscious feeling that she must do right, that her purposes toward right conduct are fixed. It is expected that she has a fairly well-developed conscience which will help to guide her into right-doing. Why should she try to do right? What tests shall she apply to her conduct to see if it is right, when she is in doubt?

The Real Test of Right Conduct is Social Welfare, the Good of All Concerned.—Social well-being is the great law under which our lives must be lived, if we would live rightly. If, when we are in doubt, we pause long enough to honestly ask ourselves what effect on general welfare would be produced if every one did this or that thing which we are doing, considering, or desiring, we will begin to get some light on the question that will show us how we should proceed.

Truthfulness.—Is truthfulness an absolute duty? To this there can hardly be more than one answer; yet a nurse is seldom very long in a hospital before she learns that to tell the truth promiscuously to every one who chooses to pry into affairs, which often are really not his concern, would lead to disastrous results to herself and to others. Are we under obligation to tell the truth to any one who chooses to ask it? We quickly learn that there are individual rights which should always be held precious. We learn that there is a field in which those inquiring have a right to the truth, a field in which individuals repose mutual confidence in each other, and where nothing but truth should be considered, yet even in this field much judgment in telling the truth is required. Plain truth in many circumstances amounts to practical falsehood, since it often conveys a wrong impression. A well-known writer* states this point admirably in the following illustration:

"When a patient who has the earliest recognizable signs of phthisis in one lung, and tubercle bacilli in his sputum, asks, 'Have I got consumption?' it would be conveying a false impression to say, 'Yes, you have,' and stop there. Ten to one his impression is that by consumption I mean a disease invariably and rapidly fatal. But this is not at all my impression of his case. To be true to the patient one must explain that what he means by consumption is the later stages of a neglected or unrecognized disease; that some people have as much trouble as he now has and get over it without finding it out; that with climatic and hygienic treatment he has a good chance of recovery, etc. To tell him simply that he has consumption without adding any further explanation would convey an impression which in one sense is true, in the sense, namely, that to another physician it might sound approximately correct. What is sometimes called the simple truth, the 'bald truth,' or the 'naked truth,' is often practically false. It needs to be explained, supplemented, modified."

Is a Lie Ever Excusable?—A question that is sometimes asked is whether, in nursing, a lie is excusable when it is told solely for the patient's benefit and without any selfish motive on your part. From time immemorial this sort of lie has been cited as excusable when

* Dr. Richard Cabot.

dealing with the sick. This question will be discussed more fully later on. In the beginning of a nurse's career, where there is any doubt as to whether the full truth should be told, there is always provided the protecting rule for the pupil, that the head nurse, or house doctor, visiting physician, or superintendent is the one who should give out information concerning the patient's condition to his friends. It is clearly not the pupil nurse's business or responsibility to deal with this matter, which she cannot fully understand. It would be folly, however, to prohibit a nurse from saying with gladness when occasion arises, "The patient is feeling much better." When dealing with those outside the circle of the patient's family or friends, a pupil nurse can always protect herself by the statement of the rule which generally exists in hospitals: "We are not allowed to give out information about our patients." The important question is not always, "Should I tell the truth or tell an untruth," but very often it is, "Is it necessary to tell anything at all at this time?" There is an old saying that "You are rarely or never sorry for the things you did not say," and it is well worth remembering by pupil nurses. It will be readily seen that truth-telling, even in the realm where others have right to the truth, is a matter that requires much judgment, and that the way the truth is told counts tremendously in its effects.

In telling the truth in a hospital there is another side to the question which admits of little argument. It is clear that a nurse who attempts to keep back the truth from the doctor or from those in charge in the hospital is a dangerous element and an unfit person to have charge of the sick. The medical treatment of a patient depends very largely on the statements of the nurse as to his condition. The doctor sees his patient but a few minutes each day and naturally and properly depends on those who have the patient under their observation and care constantly to give him an exact and true report of things as they are. Omitting to tell the whole truth, or suppressing important facts or happenings, which should be told, is deceiving those who have a right to know, and is inexcusable. No hospital can afford to tolerate such practices.

Truth in Nursing Reports.—Similarly, a nurse's reports to the head nurse or house physician, and her written records, should be as free from exaggeration, from evasion or deceit in any form, as she can possibly make them. Proper nursing, proper medical treatment, can be built only on a foundation of absolute truth as far as truth is known. Mistakes may occur, but should be promptly and honestly confessed to those who have a right to know, and who are in a position to correct them or to lessen the bad results of mistakes. Inexactness in speech, half truths, the covering up accidents or mistakes, all, in course of time, react on the nurse in ways she does not understand. How can a nurse expect a hospital to recommend her for any important position, if she leaves in the institution a record of deceit, or of attempts to deceive those in authority? No nurse ever does deceive those in authority very long, though she may think she does.

Discreetness of Speech.—Many centuries ago an ancient writer spoke of the tongue as an unruly member, and time has not changed its habits. A large part of the training for which a nurse must be responsible in herself is the training of her tongue, the cultivation in herself of habits of reticence, habits of refraining from discussing the affairs of patients with people who have no right to be told anything about them, of refraining from discussing with patients matters with which they have no concern and which she often does not fully understand. Endless trouble, untold hours of agony have been caused by the thoughtless habit of some nurse talking with patients about things of which she herself has little real knowledge.

A doctor leaves an order for a patient to be prepared for an important operation. The nurse while making the preparations remarks that "most of the patients who have had this operation have had cancer." The patient immediately and naturally wonders if she too has cancer and if the doctor has deceived her. Her anxiety is quickly communicated to her friends and to the doctor. He comes to the principal to know who told his patient she had cancer, and a general fuss follows this apparently innocent but terribly unwise and wholly unnecessary remark which the nurse made. This is one illustration of thousands which most hospitals can furnish of the trouble caused by nurses who allow their tongues to run wild, who talk at random about vital matters of which they know very little that is definite and on subjects which are better avoided.

A patient asks a nurse if she knows what was done in the operation she has just undergone. The nurse has seen stated on the operating-room records that the appendix was removed, and she states just what she had read on the records. She tells the truth. The patient had convinced herself that she would never be well till appendix and some other parts of her anatomy were removed, and she begins to worry. She censures the surgeon when he comes for not doing all that she was sure was needed. The doctor inquires how she knows what was done, and here follows another general disturbance, wholly unnecessary.

The Talkative Nurse.—The nurse who has brought with her a predisposition to "tell things" which are better untold is one of the great problems of hospital life. How to deal with her, whether such nurses should ever be allowed to finish a nursing course, is one of the great unsettled questions. It rests entirely with the nurse herself whether she becomes this sort of problem in a hospital or not. She herself is the one who must learn to control her tongue. No one else can do it. Does a nurse really desire to be recommended as "a safe woman to be admitted into one's confidence?" Let her learn to manage the little unruly member. Let her cultivate every day the habit of not telling things which need not be told, however great the temptation may be.

Telling One's Friends.—Nurses frequently think that they may tell anything they choose about their patients to their own personal friends or members of their own family, or to other nurses. Are they right or wrong in so interpreting their duties? Should a nurse in training who gossips with her friends outside the hospital about hospital patients ever be allowed to graduate? A well-known, wealthy lady entered a hospital for her first confinement. One foot of the baby was slightly bent, requiring only a little manipulation to straighten it. One of the nurses on duty told a married nurse friend of hers that the baby had a club-foot. Of course she thought her nurse friend would not tell, but the people concerned were prominent and the story was quickly told. It spread to the circle of the patient's friends and lost nothing in the telling. Several friends came to the doctor to inquire if anything could be done for the club-feet of Mrs. Blank's baby. The story was traced back to the home of the married nurse who encouraged pupils to bring all the gossip of the hospital to her.

What course should training-school authorities follow to try to stamp out this habit of gossiping about patients' affairs outside the hospital?

Rash accusations and hasty judgments are failings that are not confined to nurses, but against which nurses should guard. A nurse on night duty misses her watch and immediately, when a general search fails to bring it to light, concludes that it has been stolen. She suspects that one of the men servants took it. Before reporting the matter to the principal she informs the police. The suspected servant is placed under surveillance. A few days later the nurse finds the watch under the mattress on her bed where she herself had placed it. What harm has been done by her hasty judgment, her readiness to cast suspicion? What can be done to undo the results of her mistake? How will this mistake affect the estimate of other people regarding the nurse in question? What, in your judgment, should the authorities of the hospital do in regard to such an occurrence?

Suggestions for Written Work.—Prepare a series of not less than ten Do's and Don'ts for nurses in regard to truthfulness and to the wise use of the tongue as it relates to nursing.

QUESTIONS FOR DISCUSSION OR REVIEW

1. What tests may a nurse apply to her conduct to be sure that it is right?

2. How far should we speak the truth concerning our patients?

3. What limitations should a nurse place on herself when asked for information concerning a patient's condition?

4. What ethical principle does a nurse violate when

she gives to others information which has come to her because of her work as a nurse?

5. Mention some reasons why an untruthful nurse should not be retained in a hospital school.

6. How does the fact of inexactness or deceit in speech affect the estimate which others place on a nurse?

7. How may inexactness in speech affect a nurse's success professionally? Financially?

8. In what way may a nurse's records affect the general course of treatment prescribed for a patient?

CHAPTER VI

Old-fashioned Virtues (*Continued*)

The conception which an individual holds as to his duty is an important index to his character. What does duty mean? Webster defines duty as "that which a person is bound by moral obligation to do or refrain from doing; that which one ought to do; service that is morally obligatory." Duty is a graver term than obligation. It implies, in some cases, obedience or submission to superiors in authority.

Duty to God implies reverence, worship and loving obedience. Duty to ourselves implies temperance, courage, self-respect, and due attention to our own health and well-being. Duty to others implies absolute justice, charitable judgment, and helpful service as we have opportunity and they have need.

The Sense of Duty.—Even a very superficial study of a group of people will show that the sense of duty is much stronger in some individuals than others. One person sees what seems to be a duty of common humanity, and is impelled to perform it. Another sees the same thing, but has no feeling that he has any moral obligation to concern himself in any way about it. Ability to help plays a large part in determining our duty. Does our sense of duty depend to any extent on our early training and environment? Is it true that in the performance of that which has been generally agreed to be a duty there is often a curious mixture of motives such as pride, sympathy, love of approval or applause, regard for public opinion, fear of external consequences, or hope of material reward? Give an example from your own experience that illustrates this point. Is our sense of duty strengthened or weakened according to the ideals of life which we have before us?

Obedience.—One of the first lessons a child learns in the home is the lesson of obedience to those who naturally have authority over him. When he goes to school he has the duty of obdience still further impressed upon him, until, when he reaches the age when he can reason things out for himself, he should be able to see that obedience and respect for authority are fundamental to real success in practically any field of activity he may choose to enter. In the hospital these virtues assume an importance that cannot be overestimated. Does obedience in the hospital and obedience in the home mean exactly the same thing? Not altogether. In the home there is less necessity for the strict enforcement of obedience in matters of time, and in various other ways. Timeliness and punctuality are closely related to obedience in the hospital.

To learn to do the thing ordered punctually, when she is busy, when her own judgment opposes it or when she feels it to be unnecessary; to refrain from arguing the case when she feels she has a strong side to present; to make no grumbling comments about the order; to grasp the thought that the thing ordered is to be done even if it be inconvenient and so difficult as to be well-nigh impossible—these are qualities to be coveted and cultivated in every nurse. To make for herself a reputation for being faithful and dependable is possible for every nurse, even in her probation period, and this sort of reputation means much all through the training. It means still more in the years to come.

Be a probationer never so clever in examinations, alert, and skilful, she will be a failure as a nurse if she fails to observe the rules of those in authority, and if she omits or neglects things ordered which she did not find it convenient to do. Every hospital wants nurses who will do the thing ordered, at the proper time if at all possible, and if they find it impossible to carry out an order they will at once report it to those responsible for having that duty done. Exceptions to this rule may be necessary if a patient's condition changes so that the reason for the order being given has passed or there is need of some modification. Even then these matters should be reported to those in charge.

The quality of being teachable is one of the most important that a nurse has to cultivate, not only at the beginning but all through her nursing career. No one admires an unteachable nurse, or a nurse who is confident that she knows more than she really does. In the beginning it is not of material consequence that a nurse know anything about nursing; the important thing is whether she is capable of learning and eager to do so. She will probably have to unlearn much that she already knows or thinks she knows, and to be taught many duties in which she already feels proficient. This is a part of the daily discipline which goes on unconsciously and which has such a large part in the real training process.

Attitude under Reproof.—The attitude assumed by nurses under reproof affects greatly their own happiness and the harmony of the school. Nurses are mistaken when they regard themselves as isolated units or when they try to deceive themselves into thinking that their manners or methods affect only themselves. The nurse who is sullen or defiant when she is shown her mistakes and what she must do to correct them constitutes a real problem in every school. Too often, instead of accepting rebuke and caution with meekness and with singleness of heart, deciding that she will give no further occasion for correction on that point, she goes about clamoring for sympathy, proclaiming to other nurses "that she is tired of being scolded," or that someone "has a pick on her," and indulges in self-pity that is always unwholesome.

Minor offenses can easily become major offenses in a training school, by the attitude of the nurse concerned when she is rebuked. It is a minor offense if a nurse leaves certain utensils, for which she is responsible, in a soiled condition when she goes off duty. If, however, when the nurse is recalled to properly care for those utensils she refuses to do it, the offense assumes an entirely different aspect. A major offense has been created by the nurse out of a minor offense, and the major offense strikes at the very foundations of the discipline in the school. The first offense is readily understood and is excusable. The larger offense growing out of it is inexcusable.

Lack of respect for authority is a distinctive mark of bad breeding and stamps a nurse as undisciplined and defective in her conception of her real place in the institution. Lack of respect is frequently shown in the use of slang terms when applied to doctors or to those in authority. The use of slang shows that the nurse is lacking in true culture and in her sense of what is right and proper; it reflects on the home training which she has received.

Discipline is a term of which a nurse hears much, and

in a general way she learns a good deal about it without trying to. To the young nurse the need for strict discipline is not always apparent. Quite often she resents it because she has a wrong idea of its value. Discipline has been defined as "the difference between an army and a mob." One writing on this subject has said: "Discipline in its best sense means to educate, and to educate is to bring out of yourself your very best abilities in orderly fashion. There is no lost motion in the action of a well-disciplined army. Every move counts. The wonder of any of our great modern business enterprises is its smooth-working discipline. Maximum power demands maximum discipline. To discipline your will, your emotions, your desires is no easy job. To some it is a tremendous task, but to the man who through patient and determined effort finally brings his every ability into control and harmony, there is created a momentum that makes the greatest works come easy, all of which is the result of discipline."

In a hospital a system of semi-military discipline prevails. The rules, regulations and orders are as a rule passed to nurses through officers or workers higher in rank. The nurse is expected to observe the orders and rules given to those to whom authority has been delegated, whatever her personal feeling toward the individual may be. Each worker is expected to be in his own place until relieved from duty; to attend to the responsibilities assigned to him and not to interfere with the duties or affairs of others. Only thus can a general hope to command an army successfully. Only thus can an institution achieve its highest success. These rules do not prevent a spirit of helpfulness to each other; they do not hinder, for instance, one nurse in the same ward or corridor whose work is finished helping another who is delayed in getting through; they do prevent nurses from assuming responsibilities promiscuously and, perhaps with the best of intentions, doing harm. It may seem a small thing for a nurse or probationer to give a patient not in her charge, who calls to her, a glass of water, yet there are occasions when to give even a glass of water may be harmful to a patient, and for that reason she must go to those in charge of the patient and ask about it before doing it.

Laxity in discipline in a training school is always a detriment to the nurses, even though they may think it a desirable thing. A free and easy manner among nurses while on duty, a failure on the part of those in charge of the departments to properly enforce rules made for the good of all concerned, is an indication of slip-shod work, and an attitude of carelessness that bodes no good to the institution or to the nurses in training. No one, as a rule, is thankful for strict discipline while undergoing it. It is only appreciated when, after experience is gained, we are in a position to contrast a well-disciplined school with the other kind, and to compare the results as shown in nurses' habits, spirit and ideals.

Rules and regulations in a hospital are the outgrowth of experience and conditions. They are at once a means of education and of promoting the comfort and general welfare of all connected with the hospital. Without rules, any individual is at liberty to impose on others, and disorder, discomfort and lack of harmony are the result. Not every nurse in a hospital needs all the existing rules, but it is safe to say that unless conditions had arisen to make each rule necessary, it would not have been made. It may seem irksome at first to have a rule specifying the time that lights must be out and nurses in bed, but experience clearly proves the necessity for it. To have a rule that nurses must clean the bath tub after using it seems trivial, even humiliating—one feels like apologizing for it—yet a little observation shows that even girls from good homes have neglected this homely and necessary duty, until they were reminded that it was a rule. In their final effect rules are educative, and the keeping of them an important part of one's training. Instead of thinking of rules as irksome, they should be regarded as guide posts on the path of duty, necessary measures designed to promote the general good.

Credulity is defined as readiness to believe on slight evidence. Because many pupils enter hospital schools with an overstock of credulity, most schools have taken some steps to protect such nurses from dangers which are well understood in every hospital. It is because of this that rules are sometimes made regarding nurses going out with men patients who have been in the hospital. Restrictions or rules in this matter should be regarded as safeguards to a nurse. They are a part of the moral safety movement in which many of the best men and women are engaged. It is surely no kindness to a nurse to allow her to be imposed on by men of uncertain character.

It is well for nurses to remember that superintendents of hospitals and principals of training schools really desire pupil nurses to have all the legitimate pleasures that are compatible with their own best interests and the highest good of the school. Many years of experience are behind each rule.

Loyalty, that indefinable quality which every institution desires in the members of its working force, is in no way better shown than by careful observance of the rules and regulations. It is, of course, shown in numerous other ways, some of which will be discussed later, but loyalty begins with careful observance of rules, even if the nurse does not understand the reason for them. If a nurse ever expects to reach a position where she will command and instruct others, she must show her fitness for such responsibility by loyalty to the school and its rules, and to those in authority.

The question of loyalty to another nurse, or loyalty to the patient and the institution, is one which a nurse frequently has to decide. What should a nurse do when a patient complains in her presence about some other nurse who is assisting in nursing the complaining patient?

Suggested Subjects for Written Work.—A nurse on night duty leaves the bed of a paralytic patient in a soiled condition when she goes off duty. Her attention is called to it, but a few days later the same thing occurs. She is sent for to change the bed and leave the patient in proper condition but refuses to come. In what necessary qualities is this nurse deficient? What disciplinary measures should the authorities of the school assume toward a nurse who manifests this defiant attitude?

FOR DISCUSSION OR REVIEW

1. Explain what you mean by the term "duty."
2. Outline briefly what you conceive to be one's duty to God, to one's own self, to others.
3. Show that in performing one's duty one may have a curious mixture of motives.
4. In what way does the matter of punctuality enter into the question of obedience?

5. Mention several ways in which a nurse's attitude under reproof may affect the happiness of others and the harmony of the school.

6. Show how major offenses may grow from very small causes in a hospital.

7. Write a short paper on discipline in a hospital showing why you believe it is important to the happiness and welfare of the hospital household.

8. What should a nurse do when a male patient, of whose character she knows practically nothing, begins to flatter her and assert his undying devotion to her?

CHAPTER VII

Putting Principles into Practice

A college president, on assuming the duties of a new position, in discussing the subject of educational ideals expressed himself as follows, and the remarks apply equally well to hospital students: "No matter how many courses you may give a student, no matter how many subjects he may study, no matter how many years he may go to school and college, or what degrees he may earn, unless you make a Christian gentleman out of him, unless he is trained to honesty, to honor, to love of truth and hatred of a lie, his education is a failure. We have been in danger of paying so much attention to the curriculum that we have lost sight of the importance of character."

In a hospital many questions of honesty and honor will present themselves to nurses—matters which they have never before had to consider. It is probable that in every life the keeping of the ten commandments and the great commandment at times presents difficulties, and nurses are no exceptions. What are the commandments from which a nurse in a hospital is most likely to be tempted to deviate? Think the matter over. Thou shalt not steal. Thou shalt not bear false witness. Thou shalt remember the Sabbath day to keep it holy. Does the keeping of any of these commandments present any special difficulty to nurses in a hospital? If so, how?

Common Honesty.—One of the difficult points for many nurses to grasp is that there is an ethical principle, a question of honor, a principle of right or wrong, involved in the smallest transaction. It is not always possible, nor should it be necessary for a nurse to have this pointed out to her by others, and it devolves upon herself to pause long enough before indulging in something questionable to ask herself whether she can justify herself in doing it, whether she is being true to her best self in pursuing a certain course, whether she will lessen her own self-respect by so doing. Strange as it may seem, the practice of common everyday honesty is the point at which many nurses fail. They apparently do not mean to be dishonest, but their consciences are either too undeveloped to perceive when a thing is honest and when it is dishonest, or they deliberately violate clearly accepted ethical principles of guidance that a child of ten ought to know should be observed for the common good of all.

Is it honest or is it not for nurses on duty to use sugar supplied to the wards for the use of patients in making fudge for their own use? Is it honest or not for nurses to look into letters belonging to others? Is it honest or not for nurses to write letters to friends on temperature charts or record blanks belonging to the hospital? Is it honest or not for a nurse to nibble at the fruit in the ice-box which has been brought to some patient by his friends? Is it honest or not for a nurse to use for herself delicacies provided by the hospital especially for patients? Is it honest or not for a nurse to say on her application blank that she will, if admitted, observe the rules of the institution, then violate them deliberately and say nothing about it to those in charge? Thus illustrations might be multiplied, of practical ethical questions which a nurse will have presented to her in the daily routine, questions in which there is an important ethical principle involved. The way in which she decides such questions affects not only herself but the whole tone of the school, and often the reputation of the hospital. Few more humiliating experiences come to a principal or head nurse than to have to confess to a patient that fruit or delicacies brought to him which he could not use at the time have mysteriously disappeared; yet such an occurrence is not so unusual as one might wish, and drastic measures have had to be taken in some hospitals to prevent this very thing occurring. Petty dishonesty is contagious, so is high-principled, through-and-through honesty. It remains for every nurse to decide which sort of influence she will exert.

The question of her rights may be suggested. A nurse's rights are those which may freely be accorded to every other nurse in the institution, those and no more. No hospital can afford to have favorites, to grant certain nurses privileges to indulge in practices which it would forbid in others. The harmony and good feeling so desirable in a hospital must be based on equal justice to all.

A Nurse's Honor.—A high sense of honor is one of the best things which a nurse can bring with her to any school or to any work in which she may, later on, engage. It is difficult to analyze the elements of this intangible thing called honor, but every nurse understands to a greater or less degree what it means. It is defined as "a keen sense of what is right, just, and true, with the course of life corresponding thereto; or as strict conformity to the duty imposed by conscience, position or privilege; or as a scrupulous regard for integrity and reputation."

Integrity, that spirit of whole-hearted honesty, which excludes all forms of injustice that might favor one's self, has special reference to uprightness in mutual dealings, to the carrying out of trusts for others, and to those matters which rules and laws cannot reach or enforce. It is especially in matters which cannot well be reached by laws or rules that a nurse's sense of honor will be tested, in the carrying out of obligations in the right way, even though no one but the nurse herself may ever know of the matter which involved the question of honor. To be true to one's self, to one's own best ideals, is the hardest task a nurse will ever undertake.

> "To thine own self be true.
> And it must follow as the night the day,
> Thou canst not then be false to any man."

might fittingly be chosen as a motto for a school, a class, or a life.

Carrying out the letter of a law or rule, but deliberately violating the spirit of it, is a temptation which comes to every nurse at some time. It is one which involves, directly, the nurse's personal sense of honor. To do a thing or to refrain from doing it, simply because one is trusted, is a real test of character. The thing in itself may seem unimportant but the principle involved is tremendously important to every nurse.

This fine sense of honor which a nurse possesses, or fails to possess, is one of the great factors in her success after graduation. Where it is absent, where the nurse has shown herself lacking in this characteristic, recommendations, if given at all, are often given reluctantly. The one from whom the recommendation is sought is not quite confident how the nurse will meet the character tests of the new position which she seeks, though technically she may be fully qualified. The recommendation is therefore given, if at all, with reservations. The sense of honor is frequently the intangible quantity which decides the question between two candidates, who otherwise seem equally well qualified. The sense of honor exhibited in a thousand small ways stamps its possessor as a woman of distinctly higher grade. It is frequently in small ways where questions of honor are involved that nurses unconsciously determine their own status in nursing affairs.

The custom of nurses taking money from the sick in return for extra service rendered to them was one of the intolerable abuses in the days before trained nursing began. One of the important and sweeping reforms that followed as a result of Florence Nightingale's work and ideals for nurses was the abolition of this custom. Nurses of today occasionally are confronted with this old temptation to accept money from patients, while all reputable training schools have stringent rules against the practice. To illustrate: A young Jewess, who had been operated on, suffered most severely from thirst following operation. She had grown up with the idea that money could procure practically any sort of service that she desired for herself. She saw no reason why she might not bribe the nurse into giving her a drink of ice-water, so offered the nurse a dollar for a drink. The nurse hesitated, but finally took the money. After taking it she became afraid of it being found out that she had given the drink, kept delaying the giving of it, and finally went off duty without doing it. The patient was angry and told the head nurse of the affair. How should such an occurrence be dealt with by training school authorities, in order to impress other nurses with the seriousness of the offense? If the money had been offered for special attention instead of for the drink, would the offense have been less serious?

A young husband whose wife is to be operated on wishes as much attention as possible, without the expense of a special nurse for his wife. The head nurse in charge is young and inexperienced and he approaches her, telling her that he will "make it worth her while" to devote special attention to his wife. He begins by offering theatre tickets to the head nurse, and the day nurse in charge of his wife. Should the tickets be accepted? How should this situation be handled with the nurses? With the young husband?

In a certain school there were rigid rules against nurses taking money from patients, but small gifts from "grateful patients" were permitted. One certain nurse seemed to be extremely popular and received many more gifts than other nurses. It finally became known to other nurses that she was in the habit of dropping hints to patients as to things which she especially desired. She would proceed in some such manner as the following: After a trip to the shopping district she would remark, "I saw just the loveliest pair of dancing slippers today, just my size, number four, and only $3.50. Blank and company are having a sale. They were beauties, regular $5.00 slippers, but I hadn't enough money with me to get them; I couldn't afford them anyway, but I wanted them so much." Forthwith a pair of the bargain sale dancing slippers are secured for the nurse by the "grateful patient." Or she would remark, "I'll be so glad when I am earning something. I'm just crazy to have one of those new shopping bags; my old one is so shabby; but of course a nurse in training has to go without such luxuries. Three years seems an awful long time not to be earning anything," and the shopping bag would be presented by the next patient. What should nurses do who discover that one of the pupil nurses is inviting gifts to herself in this manner? What effect would the general practice of this custom by all nurses have on the tone and general reputation of the school? How would it be likely to affect a graduate nurse's methods later in life; in private or institutional work? What measures should be used in regard to it?

Honest confession of accidents or mistakes made or of neglect, whether intentional or unintentional, is one of the finest indications that a nurse can give that she is possessed of those high principles of conduct that should characterize a nurse. Honest confession creates in the minds of those in charge of the school a feeling of confidence in a nurse and respect for her character, that will linger in their memories long after training days are past.

This principle is probably nowhere so frequently violated in a school as in the matter of breakage of hospital appliances. The cost of the article concerned may be small, but the principle involved is far from small. It seems difficult to understand the habit of concealment or denial of knowledge of how the article came to be broken or destroyed, which many nurses show in their daily life. It is difficult to understand how they regard the whole matter, or why they are willing to violate their conscientious principles for the sake of the small sums involved. What can one high-principled nurse do to quicken the consciences of her associates who are given to denial or concealment in such matters?

The Rights of Others.—Occasionally a nurse is found whose home training has been so defective that she has little or no regard for the rights and property of others. Such nurses will borrow, without asking, articles of clothing belonging to other nurses and wear them and be deeply indignant when they are complained of, or are taken to task for such breaches of conduct. They will loudly insist on the innocence of their intentions when called to account, yet seem utterly unable to see that because another nurse is a friend, or is sharing the same room, it does not give them the right to appropriate her property. They would scorn to take money, but have no scruples about taking such articles as stockings or gloves, wearing them out, and never replacing them.

Borrowing money from other nurses with no prospect of paying for years is another questionable proceeding frequently indulged in by nurses in training. Many college students are obliged to borrow money to tide them through their period of training, and the same is true of hospital students. But borrowing small sums of money promiscuously from other nurses is certain to create difficulties for the one who borrows and for the one who loans. It is no disgrace to have to borrow money, but the way in which the borrowing is managed may be disgraceful, and the things for which nurses borrow money are often exceedingly ridiculous. The judgment of the nurse who borrows money in order that she may give Christmas presents to her friends is certainly open to question, and many nurses have done this ridiculous thing. A nurse, known to the author, borrowed five dollars from another nurse saying she needed it to buy clothing. Instead, she used the money to secure a pretty frame for a large photograph of the gentleman who for the moment occupied the center of her affections, and with the remainder she purchased some elaborate lingerie which she certainly could have done without. Ten years after, the borrowed money was still unpaid. The nurse who needs a loan of money to tide her over till she becomes an earner should frankly go to the principal of the school and talk matters over. There are dignified and proper ways of securing such loans without embarrassing one's associates by asking for the loan of money which they themselves need.

The practice of honesty enters every day into such matters as the taking of temperatures and of making records and the most severe tests of character often come in the doing of routine duties.

A nurse who was on night duty had the care of the patients on one floor. Most of these patients were children who were undergoing orthopedic treatment. As a rule none of the orthopedic patients were kept in this ward for more than two weeks to a month. A part of her duty was to take the temperatures of the children in this ward every morning. This became a tedious duty. In many of the children there was little or no change in temperature from morning to morning, so she decided to omit taking the temperatures of children who showed little variation, and simply mark the charts each morning as though she had taken the temperatures. What ethical principles did she violate in so doing? How would you characterize this offense?

A nurse hated sponging typhoid fever patients. There was a standing order that all such patients should be sponged if the temperature went above 102°F. It became known that when this certain nurse was on duty the temperatures of fever patients were rarely recorded above 102°F. She either did not leave the thermometer with the patient long enough to secure a proper record, or she deliberately falsified the records of the temperatures and marked the charts always below the sponging point. What effect would this practice have on the work of the hospital if commonly indulged in? How can a principal prevent such breaches of trust on the part of nurses? What disciplinary measures should be used with nurses who fall under this temptation?

Suggested Subject for Written Work.—A nurse is in charge of a patient with a very poor appetite. The doctor allows the patient to have ice cream whenever she wishes, and a small freezer containing a quart is ordered daily to be sent to the diet kitchen to be used especially for this patient. Soon after the first supply is sent to the diet kitchen, the nurse in charge is seen secretly treating two other nurses to ice cream from this patient's supply. What qualities of character are shown in this transaction, by the nurse in charge of the patient, by the other two nurses? How would this and similar practices affect the hospital, the nurse herself, and the tone of the school? What measures should be taken to check such practices? What attitude should the authorities assume toward nurses who persistently indulge in such practices in spite of admonition?

FOR DISCUSSION OR REVIEW

1. Mention those parts of the ten commandments which seem to furnish special difficulties to nurses.
2. What do you mean by "a sense of honor?"
3. Show how the possession of a keen sense of honor may be a help to a nurse when seeking a position.
4. Give some reasons why the custom of nurses taking money from patients should not be tolerated in a hospital.
5. What is the difference in principle between taking money and taking other gifts?
6. Should the accepting from patients of small favors or other gifts be permitted among nurses in a hospital? Give reasons for your answer.
7. What method should be followed when every nurse on a floor denies breaking an article, which one nurse must have broken?
8. Show how the principle of honesty enters into the taking of temperatures and the keeping of records.

CHAPTER VIII

Ethics and Economy

Economy and efficiency are two important goals which hospitals try to keep before them in their management. Economy without efficiency in the care of the sick is hardly creditable. Efficiency without economy is indicative of ignorance and poor management.

"Economy," says Webster, "is management without loss or waste; prudence, with a disposition to save. Economy avoids waste and extravagance and applies money to the best advantage. Frugality cuts off ordinary indulgences, and insists on systematic saving. The latter conveys the idea of not using or spending superfluously, and is opposed to lavishness or profusion. Parsimony is frugality carried to extremes, involving meanness of spirit and a sordid mode of living. Economy is a virtue, and parsimony a vice." It will thus be seen that a virtue when carried to extremes may become a vice, and that wise judgment is needed in a hospital to know where to draw the dividing line.

Most hospitals have some rules of guidance for nurses in these matters. The rule that commonly exists, that worn linen or defective appliances are not to be cast aside, but should be brought in exchange for new articles of the same kind, is a wise rule that tends to economy and relieves nurses of the necessity of deciding when a thing is of no further use.

Another rule that should be unnecessary is that towels,

pillow covers, and such things shall be used for the purposes for which they are intended and for no other; this has prevented some careless nurses from using them as dusters or cleaning cloths. Rules that ice-caps or hot-water bottles must not be placed in coverings which are pinned with common pins have saved such articles from being promptly punctured by heedless nurses. But with all the safeguards that hospital workers have been able to devise to prevent thoughtless damage and waste by nurses, there is still much room for the individual nurse to exercise her judgment and to help or hinder the hospital in using the money entrusted to it to the very best advantage.

The Handling of Hospital Property.—Many nurses who have been accustomed to the freedom of a home find it exceedingly difficult to get the thought fixed in their "inner consciences" that the hospital supplies and property which they are handling do not belong to them, that their rightful use is limited to that which is actually needed for those persons for whom the supplies were intended.

Is it Wrong to be Wasteful?—This question admits of little argument. Waste, as a general rule, indicates either ignorance or lack of conscience in the person responsible. Yet wilful extravagance on the part of nurses is not unusual. Many nurses have the mistaken idea that because the property belongs to the city or to a corporation it makes little or no difference to anyone whether they are careless or extravagant or not in the way they handle supplies in their department. "Use all you want to, the city pays for it," or "we don't have to pay for it" are remarks frequently heard that are indicative of the attitude of some nurses, especially in larger institutions.

Free Service.—Two important sides to this question should be carefully considered by every nurse. Whether the hospital is supported from taxpayers' money as a municipal institution, or whether from funds entrusted to the board of managers by private individuals to be used for the benefit of the sick, the fact remains that the work of every hospital is affected in quality or quantity by the amount of money it has to spend, and this is especially true in relation to its charity. Most hospitals have as many free beds as possible with the money at their disposal. The cost of keeping up a free bed in an average American hospital will probably be found to be somewhere between $1.75 and $2.75 a day, the higher figure depending on a variety of things—proportion of ward patients, a busy accident service, expensive laboratory and research departments, and other items, the cost varying each year with the general cost of living.

What is meant by a free bed is that it is free to the occupant, that someone else pays the cost. Most hospitals desire to provide for the sick poor as much free care as possible with limited funds. Thus it is easily seen that waste, just small waste, of milk, soap, gauze, absorbent cotton, electric light, gas, breakage which should have been prevented, each nurse wasting a little of these and other articles every day, mounts up in a year to much larger sums than nurses are aware of. It lessens considerably the service the hospital is able to render to the sick poor. This is one serious side to the matter of waste, or carelessness, in the use and care of hospital supplies and appliances.

Extravagance in nurses has another serious side which relates to the nurse herself. Habits of waste or carelessness, of extravagance, are a decided hindrance to a nurse's success as a private or institutional nurse. They are defects of character which quickly show up and make her undesirable as a worker. A wasteful, extravagant or careless head nurse is not a safe example for pupil nurses; therefore few institutions desire to keep such nurses in positions of responsibility. An extravagant or careless private nurse is too expensive a commodity for most private households, and her reputation for these habits soon spreads.

"We could have paid the trained nurse her regular charges by going in debt, but we found after a few days that she was so extravagant in different ways that we couldn't afford to keep her, so we let her go and got an untrained woman who could get along with less and who knew something about economy." This bit of real conversation shows how the habits which a nurse forms while in training may quickly affect her professional reputation and her financial success as an independent worker. How does a nurse acquire such habits? To some extent they are acquired before she comes to the training school. Nurses are inclined to be either careful or careless, to be economical or the opposite, before they ever see inside a training school. Part of the practice of carelessness or extravagance is due to sheer thoughtlessness; part is due to a wrong attitude of mind toward the whole problem; part is due to not knowing the cost of various articles and how the waste or carelessness of one nurse, when multiplied by tens or hundreds, really affects to a great degree the good work which a hospital is able to do for those who most need its help.

Personal Responsibility.—It was stated in the opening chapter that one of the important points on which a nurse is judged is in her ability to be trusted with responsibility. Every nurse, in the way she uses or misuses hospital supplies, appliances and property, is showing whether she can be trusted with larger responsibility or not. Every nurse is, to a certain extent, a steward of hospital supplies; whether she is a trustworthy or untrustworthy steward is for her to decide. If she carried a placard around her neck saying "I am wasteful; I am careless about hospital property and expense," she would not reveal her character and habits more plainly than they are revealed in the everyday routine.

Bed Linen and Bedding.—In the care and use of bed linen and blankets there is much need for the exercise of good judgment, if waste and misuse of these supplies are to be avoided. It is easily possible to go to extremes in this matter, to not change the bed linen as often as is really needed, or to be extravagant in the use of bed linen and needlessly increase the work in the laundry, as well as add unnecessarily to the wear and tear of linen as it goes through the laundry process. An investigation as to the constant shortage of linen in a certain department of a hospital revealed the fact that some nurses changed the sheets every time they gave the patient a bath. Nurses on special duty in that department gave daily baths, as a rule, and changed the sheets daily whether they were soiled or not. Clean folded sheets were used as draw sheets, or used as pads under bed pans, and the same sort of carelessness was observed in regard to towels and other articles.

Good judgment is needed in using linen in cases where extensive wet dressings are used or in cases of burns or certain forms of skin diseases where the remedies used are of an oily nature, liable to leave an indelible stain on new linen or blankets. Likewise, also, special care is needed in regard to blankets used for baths, or for wrapping convalescents.

Common examples of the abuse of everyday appliances may serve to furnish the beginning of a list, which every nurse can add to from her own observation.

1. Scissors are used to remove corks from bottles and the points are broken.

2. Boiling drinks are poured into glass tumblers.

3. Hypodermic needles are left without wires and quickly rendered useless.

4. Thermometers are placed in the mouths of delirious patients or children and forgotten.

5. Utensil sterilizers are allowed to boil dry.

6. Glass barrel syringes are left on tables or window sills and roll off.

An excellent object lesson in what not to do with hospital appliances was shown at one of the conventions of the American Hospital Association. It consisted of a collection of articles ruined by misuse,* the articles being arranged in flat, square, cardboard boxes. The collection illustrated the following evidences of waste or misuse:

Destruction of polished woodwork by hot water, soap and alcohol.

Result of nurse splashing gown with Labarraque's solution.

Destruction of rubber by oil.

Sling used to clean ink bottles.

Burnt rectal tube.

Burning of bedding, blankets, sheets, spread, mattress, etc., by leaving 16-candle-power lamp with shade on bed for one-half hour.

Broken glass syringe.

Result of uncovered hot-water bag lying on glass-top table.

* Collection arranged by Miss Lauder Sutherland, Hartford Hospital, Hartford, Conn.

Result of boiling an infant's woolen stocking.

Result of putting rubber tubing away with clamp down.

Destruction of rubber cap by ether.

Result of using towel to wipe up tincture of iron.

Result of 16-candle-power drop-light left in contact with mirror in a dresser.

Result of steam sterilization of celluloid combs.

Result of placing silver teapot over gas flame.

Child's leather shoes spoiled by steam sterilization.

Bathroom rug with olive-oil stains.

How is Waste to be Prevented?—There is no one remedy which can be depended on to prevent waste, but much may be accomplished in this direction by systematic instruction, and by creating in the heart of each nurse a genuine desire to avoid waste. Theoretically, at least, most nurses profess to abhor waste. They will say emphatically "If there is one thing I hate it is waste," and sometimes immediately proceed to use four times the amount of gauze needed for a pad, thereby making it cost the hospital four times what it should, or they cut a bandage instead of patiently unwinding it, or they do something else diametrically opposite to wise use or economy.

Thrift.—The very first step in the promotion of thrifty habits is the taking account of the items handled in the daily routine, and their cost. A good method which is practised in some hospitals is to tabulate for each department each month the name and cost of each article broken or destroyed by misuse. These lists are distributed to the head nurses, to be by them presented to the pupils. This has the advantage of not only bringing to them the total cost of breakage each month, but of giving an opportunity for comparison between different wards

8-28-'14-2M-8

HARTFORD HOSPITAL.

Ward Requisition.

Date, April 13 1915

Ward, 9 Head Nurse, H. L. Jones

Exchange	New	NAME OF ARTICLES	Estimated Cost
	1	Gauze,	$2.25
	2	Cotton, Absorbent,	.30
	2	Cotton, Common.	.20
	24	Bandages, (2 inch)	.72
	50	Safety Pins,	.07
	1	Temperature charts	.20
	1	Daily ward report	.15
	1	Temperature book	.20
	2	Blotters	.06
	1	Roll adhesive	.80
	1	Glass pitcher	.35
	6	Orange wood sticks	.12
	500	Tongue depressors	.45
	6	Baby bottles ℥8	.18
1		Medicine glass	.03
1		Vase	10
		Total,	$6.21

Approved, ____________________ Prin. of Training School.

____________________ Superintendent.

Received by H. L. Jones ____________________ Head Nurse.

Hartford Hospital

GROCERY REQUISITION

8M.-6-3-'14

Ward 9

Date April 13-15

No. of Private Patients ——

" " Ward " 20

Bon Ami	2 cakes.	.16
Cereals, Dry		
Chocolate		
Cocoa	1 lb.	.36
Coffee	1 lb.	.24
Crackers	1 lb	.07
Flour		
Flaxseed		
Floor Wax		
Lemons		
Lime, Chloride of		
Matches	1 pkg.	.04
Mustard		
Pepper		
Powder, Gibson's		
Salt		
Sapolio		
Soap—Chips		
Laundry	4 cakes.	.14
Toilet	4 cakes	.18
Soda, Washing		
Starch		
Sugar—Granulated	4 lbs.	.20
Loaf		
Condensed milk.	3 cans.	.39
Vinegar		$1.68

A. K. Brown
Head Nurse.

Approved:

Principal of Training School.

or departments. The carelessness of workers in one department is often best appreciated when contrasted

Hartford Hospital

DIET REQUISITION

Ward 9

Date April 13-15

No. of Private Patients

" " Ward " 20

	Breakfast	Dinner	Supper
House Diet	20	20	20
Eggs	15 - .35		
Bread	1	1	1
Butter, pounds	1½ .45		
Coffee			
Beef Juice, ounces			
Toast	20	20	20
Tea			
Soup			
Cereal			
Milk, quarts	3	3	3 .63
Baby milk 11 quarts.			$1.10
Oranges	6 .02		
Lemons			
Vichy			

A. K. Brown
Head Nurse.

Ward 9.

Groceries	$1 68
Ward Supplies	3 21
Food Stuffs	20 44
Extras	
Total	$25 33
Average No. pts. 32	
Per capita cost	79

Head nurse. A K Brown

with those in a different department, where more care is exercised.

In teaching the cost of hospital supplies various methods are in use. In one hospital a collection of the common ward supplies most likely to be broken or destroyed is arranged on heavy cardboards for object teaching, the articles being fastened to the board by narrow tape. This list would include rectal nozzles and tubes, catheters, thermometers, medicine glasses, small syringes, babies' bottles, etc. The price of each article singly and by the dozen is marked. These object lessons constitute the nurse's first lessons in hospital economy. A similar method is used in another hospital where pictures of the common articles, clipped from catalogues or magazines, are mounted on sheets of cardboard with prices listed under each article. These cost demonstration boards are hung in the class room for reference and for use in teaching. Another method consists in having a price list of articles used in the wards or departments typewritten and placed in a loose-leaf book belonging to every ward. This latter system is in use in the Hartford Hospital, Hartford, Conn., and in several other hospitals, and the system is further developed by having on every requisition blank a column for costs. Specimens of these requisition blanks are shown. It should be understood that the cost of any of these articles is likely to vary from year to year and in different parts of the country.

Suggested Subject for Written Work.—Prepare a list of not less than a dozen suggestions which, if observed by nurses, would reduce cost without lowering efficiency in a hospital.

DISCUSSION OR REVIEW

1. State briefly how the question of right or wrong is related to hospital economy.

2. Give reasons why more care should be exercised in regard to hospital property than if the same were personally owned.

3. Mention several ways in which a reputation for extravagance may hinder a nurse's financial success.

4. Explain what is meant by the terms "true economy" and "false economy." Give examples of misuse or extravagance in the use of hospital linen that you have observed.

5. Mention several ways by which nurses may reduce or increase the cost of rubber goods in a hospital.

6. If one electric bulb, while burning, costs one cent for each hour, estimate the waste produced by five careless night nurses who each allowed on an average of five bulbs to burn unnecessarily for ten hours each night for a month.

7. In a certain hospital breakage is charged to the nurse responsible. Where the breakage is not admitted and the responsible person not known, the cost of the destroyed article is divided among all the nurses in the department. Is this a fair rule? Should the innocent suffer for the guilty? How should such a condition be dealt with?

8. In a surgical pavilion accommodating seventy patients, estimate the cost per patient, per day, of the gauze and cotton used in dressings.

9. State the total cost to the hospital per year of wasting an average of four inches of gauze on each patient every day, considering that the hospital had a daily average of 160 patients.

10. What should it cost to properly pad a splint eighteen inches in length and four in width?

11. Mention several examples that you have personally observed of how waste occurs in regard to surgical supplies.

12. In your own ward or department jot down the examples of waste that have come to your notice in one day.

HARTFORD HOSPITAL

Price List of Articles Used on Wards (1915.)

A

Applicators, wood, per box	0.25
Atomizer	0.30

B

Bags, hot-water	0.65
Bags, paper, T.B., per M	2.00
Bandage, Esmarch	1.00
Bandage, gauze	0.03
Basin, dressing	0.50
Basin, pus	0.50
Basket, waste	0.50
Bands, elastic, per lb	3.50
Bell	0.75
Beater, egg	0.08
Boiler, catheter	2.00
Boiler, inst	2.25
Board, chart	0.35
Blotter, small, per C	0.50
Blotter, desk	0.03
Book, patient's clothes	0.50
Book, Dr.'s order	0.25
Book, day order	0.65
Book, temperature	0.20
Bottle, baby's	0.03
Bowl, finger	0.10
Bowl, cereal	0.15
Bowl, bath	2.25
Brush, shaving	0.25
Brush, bottle	0.45
Brush, bed pan	0.50
Brush, floor	0.50
Brush, radiator	0.25
Brush, high duster	1.25
Brush, camel-hair	0.01
Brush, hair	0.20
Brush, hand	0.05
Box, sputum, tin	0.10
Box, paper, sputum, per C	0.50
Box, large, red	0.25
Box, pasteboard, T.B.	0.03½
Buckles, gross	0.50
Broom, whisk	0.25
Broom, oil	1.85
Broom, floor, corn	0.35
Bulb, electric	0.15

C

Can, clothes	2.00
Can, irrigation	0.50
Can, garbage	1.25
Can, sprinkling	0.20
Cards, morgue, per C	0.35
Cards, colored	0.01
Cap, ice	0.75
Cap, rubber	0.40
Candle	0.02
Cradle, bed	1.50
Caps, baby's bottle, gross	0.22
Catheters, silk	0.50
Catheters, rubber	0.15
Catheters, silver	0.75
Catheters, glass	0.10
Clips, large box	0.15
Clips, small box	0.08
Cots, finger, gross	0.40
Cup, feeding	0.40
Cup, drinking	0.10
Comb, large	0.50
Comb, fine-tooth	0.25

HARTFORD HOSPITAL

PRICE LIST OF ARTICLES USED ON WARDS.—(*Continued*)

Cotton, absorbent........0.15
Cotton, common.........0.10
Cushion, air.............2.25
Cup, enamel.............0.15

D

Dish, sauce..............0.10
Dish, soap, china.........0.10
Dish, soap, enamel,......0.15
Dish, square, enamel.....0.50
Depressors, tongue, M....0.90
Duster, feather...........0.75
Director, grooved........0.25

F

Funnel, enamel 0.15
Funnel, hard rubber 0.35
Funnel, glass 0.15
Forceps, sponge 1.25
Forceps, tissue 0.75
Forceps, hæmostatic.....0.75
Forks, silver, dozen......1.75
Forks, steel 0.75
File, nail 0.10

G

Glass for thermometer...0.10
Glass, drinking 0.03½
Glass, medicine 0.05
Glass, graduate, 1 pint....0.25
1 ounce 0.25
1 dram 0.25
Graduate, enamel 0.40
Glasses, eye, blue 0.10
Gauze per roll 2.25
Gloves, rubber, per pair..0.50
Gas heater 1.75

H

Hamper, clothes........2.00
Holder, match 0.40
Holder, pen 0.03
Handle, mop 0.35

I

Ink well...............0.25

J

Jar, glass, large.........2.00
Jar, surgical carriage....2.50

K

Knife, silver, dozen.....1.75
Knife, vegetable........0.15
Knife, carving..........0.75

L

Ladle, soup 0.15
Lamp, alcohol 0.25

M

Mask, eye 0.25
Medicine dropper 0.02
Mop, dish 0.10
Mop, floor 0.20
Mop, dish, wire........0.10
Mits, bath 0.25
Mugs, large and small..0.10

N

Napkins, paper, M.... 0.75
Needle, hypodermic, doz.0.75

HARTFORD HOSPITAL

Price List of Articles Used on Wards.—(*Continued*)

Article	Price
Nipple, simplex, gross	4.40
Nipple, baby welcome, gross	3.50
Nozzle, douche	0.10
P	
Pan, dust	0.25
Pan, bed, china	1.75
Pan, bed, granite	2.25
Pan, douche, granite	1.75
Pad, Kelly	7.50
Pad, scratch, pound	1.08
Pail, enamel	1.25
Pens, gross	0.40
Pencils	0.03
Paper, toilet	0.07
Paper, wrapping, pound	0.03¼
Plates, soup	0.15
Plates, dinner	0.12
Plates, breakfast	0.10
Pot, cocoa	0.40
Pot, tea, P. R. tray	1.25
Pitcher, enamel	0.75
Pitcher, glass	0.35
Pitcher, china	0.20
Plaster, adhesive	0.80
Pins, safety, gross	0.15
Pins, common, pound	0.30
Points, irrigating	0.10
Points, enema	0.10
Polisher, floor	1.75
Pump, breast	0.35
Probe, silver	0.50
Pan, sauce	0.75
Pan, sauté	0.65
R	
Razor	1.50
Ring, napkin	0.10
Ring, rubber	2.25
Ruler	0.18
Racks, baby bottle	0.25
S	
Shaker, salt	0.05
Shaker, powder	0.05
Shaker, milk	0.42
Shaker, soap	0.05
Shield, nipple	0.15
Shade, light	0.50
Saucer	0.08
Screen, four-leaf	4.00
Strainer, tea	0.10
Strainer, sink	0.35
Strainer, dish	0.50
Spoons, tea, dozen	1.00
Spoons, table, dozen	1.75
Spoons, serving	0.10
Spatula	0.22
Squeezer, glass	0.08
Sponge, desk	0.03
Sponge, bath	0.75
Strap, razor	0.60
Stick, orange	0.02
Syringe, Davidson	0.40
Syringe, glass, 1-ounce	0.35
Syringe, hard-rubber	1.25
Syringe, aural	0.25
Syringe, urethral	0.10
Syringe, hypodermic	0.30
Syringe, Sub. Q	0.60
Scissors	0.75

HARTFORD HOSPITAL

PRICE LIST OF ARTICLES USED ON WARDS.—(*Continued*)

T

Tags of all kinds, per C	0.35
Tacks, thumb, gross	1.00
Tray, pen, enamel	0.35
Tray, enamel, small	0.25
Tray, enamel, large	0.50
Tray, papier maché	0.55
Thermometer, dairy	0.25
Thermometer, bath	0.20
Thermometer, house	0.25
Tubing, rubber, pound	3.00
Tube, rectal	0.35
Tube, stomach	1.00
Tube, drink., glass, gross	1.00
Tube, drink., straw, per M.	0.33
Tube, connect., glass	0.10
Twine, ball	0.15
Tub, foot	2.25
Toothpicks	0.07
Tags, baby bottle, per M.	0.38

U

Urinal, glass	0.35
Urinal, enamel	0.30

V

Vase	0.10

W

Wringer, mop	1.75
Wires, hypodermic, bunch	0.10
Wicks, alcohol lamp	0.03

Charts

Temperature	0.23
Standing order	0.18
Laboratory report	0.15
Bedside notes	0.18
Weight	0.30
Anesthesia	0.20
Physical examination	0.50
History	0.22
Medicine, each	0.03

Pads

Short memo., pound	0.08
Death notice	0.18
Daily ward report	0.15
Critical slip	0.14
Transfer slip	0.08
X-ray slip	0.11
Pathological	0.09
Medicine	0.10
Deposit check	0.50
Nurse report	0.25
Diet requisition	0.09
D. K. requisition	0.14
Repair requisition	0.09
Emergency requisition	0.12
Grocery	0.15
Linen, green	0.13
Drug requisition	009

Groceries

Bon ami, cake	0.08
Butter, varies	0.32–0.37
Cereals, dry, pkg	0.10
Chocolate, pound	0.32
Cocoa, pound	0.36
Coffee, pound	0.24
Crackers, pound	0.07 1/5
Dust down, pound	0.01 7/8

HARTFORD HOSPITAL

Price List of Articles Used on Wards.—(*Continued*)

Eggs, dozen, varies	0.23
Flour, pound, varies	0.03
Flaxseed, pound	0.05½
Floor wax, pound	0.23
Lemons, dozen, varies	0.22
Chloride lime, pound	0.02¼
Matches, dozen boxes	0.04
Mustard, pound	0.20
Milk, quart, varies	0..05½
Oranges, dozen, varies	0.18
Pepper, pound	0.25
Gibson powder, pound	0.03¼
Salt, pound	0.01
Sapolio, cake	0.06¼
Soap chips, pound	0.06½
Soap, laundry, cake	0.03½
Soap, toilet, cake	0.02
Soda, washing, pound	0.01¾
Starch	0.03½
Sugar, granulated, pound, varies	0.05
Sugar, loaf, pound, varies	0.05½
Tea, pound	0.23
Vinegar, gallon	0.35
Condensed milk, can	0.13
Barley flour, box	0.20
Brass polish, box	0.15

CHAPTER IX

Tact and Imagination

It is hard for a nurse to realize the importance of the daily happenings which go to make up life while in the training school. It is hard for her to realize that the ethics of her personal life affect the very center of all efforts for the improvement of nurses and nursing, that what she does and is, and the influence that she is exerting, affects the whole nursing structure. Only as a school can improve the individual members of that school, can it accomplish anything in improving conditions—ethical conditions, which exist, and which rightly cause serious concern to those who have the welfare of the sick and of nurses themselves really at heart. Ethical questions are practical problems. They are questions dealing with the personal life and conduct of each nurse, with her way of looking at situations and of dealing with them as they present themselves in a more or less monotonous routine day after day. Two elements which mean much in securing the comfort of patients and the general success of the nurse are tact and imagination.

Tact is defined as the ready power of appreciating a situation, and of doing or saying that which is most suitable under the circumstances. It suggests the keenness of perception or discernment which enables a nurse to prevent awkward situations, or to avoid difficulties arising from temperamental differences. The word brings to our mind the nurse or the individual who has the happy art of keeping things running without friction, of smoothing out ruffled dispositions by a few well-chosen remarks, or by an adroit turn in the conversation.

The untactful nurse always has a difficult time. She does not get along smoothly with people. There are sharp edges to her disposition. She may be conscientious and faithful but her lack of tact prevents her from getting or keeping good positions or from making friends generally. She is very often what is called "self-opinionated," disposed to argue points when it really makes no difference, confident that she is right and that the patient or his friends, or somebody else, was wrong. She creates trouble for people in authority by her inability to smooth out minor grievances of patients and prevent them assuming larger proportions in the patient's mind. She is apt to feel that patient's likes or dislikes are of small importance. Every training school knows the untactful nurse. It is a part of the training school aim to transform untactful nurses into tactful ones, an aim not always reached. How may an untactful nurse correct this grave defect in herself? There is no one way of doing it. Two of the best methods to use are to continually and honestly try to get the viewpoint of the other person, to try to see how he looks at the matter, and to practice thinking before speaking.

A lack of sympathy with the other person is often at the bottom of a difficult situation which arises from lack of tact. A spirit of genuine everyday kindness in a nurse is quickly felt by most patients, and one does not often find troubles arising from lack of tact, where the patient is convinced of the nurse's real desire and effort to be kind. Occasionally there is encountered a grouchy person who is at odds with the world in general, and on whom kindness seems to be thrown away, but these people are exceptions. The nurse who is really kind, and who takes pains to express her kindness in such little ways as are possible to every nurse, will have comparatively little trouble in keeping her patient's dispositions from becoming seriously ruffled on her account.

Is kindness a natural or acquired gift? Can it be cultivated? If so, how? Study yourself in this matter of everyday kindness. What does it consist in?

Seeing the Real Patient.—To see the real patient we must, in most cases, try to see him or imagine him in his natural environment; we must see him in relation to his family or relatives, or, lacking these, his associates, those with whom he mingles in everyday life. We see the patient in a free bed, or we think we see him. We think he should be profoundly grateful for all that is done for him. But we frequently fail wholly in appreciating how it must feel to some natures to become dependent on the bounty of others; how it must gall and fret a man or woman of independent spirit to be obliged to occupy a free bed.

We forget that in many cases an enforced stay, even a short one, in a hospital, means loss of wages, frequently debt, worry from fear of losing a job, anxiety over family problems, perhaps overdue rent, perhaps hungry children, all these and more; yet in our shortsightedness, we see none of these things in the background, as we move in and out among the patients. We need not only good judgment but we need a kind heart, and a mind that desires keenly to understand the whole man, we need to learn to see beyond the standing orders and general routine.

In one ward we may see a man who has struggled to save to make a small payment on a little home, which will be his some day many years hence, *providing he keeps up the monthly payments* as stipulated in the contract. We can faintly imagine what loss of work, what a stay in a hospital, means in such a case.

In another bed we may see a woman for whom the joy of life has been killed because of a wayward son or daughter, or husband; in another we may see one whose whole life has been one long struggle with adversity, for whom troubles have followed fast on each other, and who looks out into the future with dread and apprehension of what it may hold for her. In a small private room, we may see a patient whose furniture has been mortgaged to secure money to tide over the illness, because she was too proud to occupy a free bed, or a bed in a general ward. We may, if we look farther, see a boy or a girl in this family who has had to give up his cherished ambition of high school or college because of the drain on the family treasury made by illness. There are so many things about our patients that we never see because we do not try to really understand them.

A clear understanding of people is rarely reached until we have learned something of what constitutes pleasure to them and what their ambitions and disappointments have been. Would we be a little more patient, a little more kind, a little more attentive to their requests, would our service be a little less mechanical, if we could see back into their lives more clearly, see each patient in his own setting, surrounded by the people and the things which make up his life? Is it part of our duty to try to see these things; to nurse the individual, not simply his disease? If so, how may we become proficient?

Imagination, the power to call up mental images, to modify our conceptions of things seen or felt, to combine different ideas so as to form new ideas in our minds, has a large place in nursing. The lack of imagination is the cause of a very great deal of dissatisfaction where nurses are concerned. The nurse who has trained her imagination and her sympathy so that she can at least dimly see things from the patient's viewpoint, will not come glibly into a patient's room and remark, "I attended my first autopsy last night," and proceed to dilate on her feelings during the autopsy and to describe the situation.

She will not come briskly into the presence of a patient with a history of pain of long standing which she fears she will have to endure till death, and inquire, "Is the pain gone this morning?" She will never tell a patient that the troubles of which he complains are imaginary, that there is nothing the matter with him if he only thought so.

She will avoid using the rocking chair when she sees it jars sensitive nerves. She will try to remember the thousand and one little things that she would like done for herself if she occupied the patient's bed. She will try to keep from a patient depressing, harrowing stories, or experiences, and to bring to him all the brightness possible.

The nurse whose imagination is developed as it should be will not permit herself to smile or to grow impatient where religious rites, ceremonies, or beliefs are concerned or mentioned. Few things are more appreciated by patients than a practical expression of sympathy with a patient in his religious belief, when he knew the nurse was not of the same belief, yet it is not uncommon to find nurses giggling or making frivolous remarks about religious observances that were tremendously important to the patient and to his friends. They did not imagine how the patient felt about it. We cannot be expected to fully understand the deep meaning embodied in all religious observances; yet we can appreciate the fact that it is an effort of the soul to link itself to the Infinite One in some way, and we can be kind, whether we understand the meaning of the symbolic rites or not.

The New Patient.—Nowhere is the lack of tact or imagination likely to cause keener suffering than in the manner shown toward new patients. To the nurse the new patient may be simply one more in the never ceasing procession of suffering or ailing individuals through the halls of pain, one more bed or room occupied, one more to carry out standing orders for, one more name to go on the diet lists. To the patient it is often a momentous experience in life, nearly always protested against and dreaded to some extent, nearly always fraught with anxiety, and more or less risk.

Standing Orders.—Apart from the standing orders for new patients which include the orders to list his clothing and put them away; send money and valuables to the office, properly marked; take temperature, pulse and respiration; give bath; make out a chart, etc., may each nurse not make out for herself a set of standing rules of ethics for new patients which might read somewhat as follows:

1. Give prompt and special attention to latest arrival in ward or department; always remember that nurses are hostesses in departments or wards, and same courtesy is required as in well-ordered home.

2. Meet friends of patient if possible and impress them with personal interest in patient.

3. Be sure to speak a few reassuring words of comfort and sympathy to patient as soon as possible after arrival. Let him know that he is going to like the hospital.

4. Find out when food was last taken. Give light nourishment if needed and permitted, and if meal is not near.

5. Inquire sympathetically about length of illness. Inquire as to whether he feels comfortable at present.

6. Find out if patient has dread of hospital, and is suffering from needless terrors, and try to remove dread.

7. Study to interpret to patient the real spirit of the institution.

8. Never ignore existence of new patient till something has to be done for him.

9. Cultivate habit of showing helpful interest, and study how to be kind as needed in each case. Try to remember likes and dislikes when special points are mentioned.

10. Remember that we are dealing with afflicted souls, hungry souls, as well as afflicted bodies.

The Patient's Friends.—In many cases the friends of patients make larger demands on us than the patients themselves. We are ready to make allowances for patients, because of illness, but are often unwilling to make allowances for the mental suffering which a patient's friends are undergoing because of his illness. Quite often the father, mother, wife or husband of a much loved patient is suffering more deeply than the patient. Soul grief, soul suffering, cuts deeper than physical suffering. For instance, a young man of good family is wounded in a quarrel, while under the influence of liquor. His father and mother and wife have worried keenly over his habits. The illness or wound may be slight or serious, but is it not entirely likely that their suffering is deeper, more acute than that of the patient?

If we have ever had a relative seriously ill we can perhaps recall our own feelings, and thus be better able to appreciate the feelings of our patient's friends.

It is never possible to make rules regarding patient's

friends that will fit all occasions that may arise, but many difficulties will be avoided if a right attitude is exhibited toward, and pleasant relations established with the friends in the beginning. First let us rid ourselves of the feeling that is far too common, that "visitors are nuisances." Let us remember that relatives and friends have some rights which we should never forget.

It is well to be guided to some extent in our dealings, not by the impression the friends make on us, but by the effect they have on the patient. A visitor may appear to us as a most unattractive and undesirable person. Her voice may be shrill, her habits noisy, and her appearance untidy. Yet to the patient she represents a familiar figure whose habits are unnoticed because of long familiarity with them, and the effect on the patient may be decidedly good; his loneliness is banished, he feels better. The visit from this most unattractive person often means more than anything we can do for him.

Visitors and Rules.—Perhaps the most difficult part of the nurse's dealings with friends of patients comes when rules have to be enforced, regarding hours when they may come, or must leave, regarding delicacies or foods forbidden, and similar necessary prohibitions.

This is a point at which nurses need tact and judgment and also a good stiff spinal column. To keep one patient's visitor from annoying other patients is a highly important duty, but when tactfully done it rarely offends. To weakly yield when in charge of a ward or corridor, and entrusted with the enforcement of rules regarding hours at which visitors should leave, and allow them to overstay their time, is no real kindness to a patient. It is a sign of lack of ability, of moral courage in a nurse. If she ever wishes to be trusted with larger responsibilities she must show herself equal to dealing with such situations.

A discerning nurse will be able to see when some visitor who has gained admittance to the patient's room is tiring the patient, and will contrive to get rid of him whether the visitor's time limit has expired or not. A difference must be recognized in dealing with the close family relatives, and with ordinary acquaintances. A great many people have a morbid desire to visit people in hospitals, who have never visited in the patient's home, and this kind of visitor is likely to prove both tiring and troublesome to deal with.

It is through the imagination that it is possible for us to put ourselves on the same plane as a child and, sympathizing with him, see things as he does, and understand in his way. Similarly we can try to put ourselves on the plane of thought and feeling which the patient occupies. We need to do this to keep from becoming mechanical in our habits of service to patients.

How shall a nurse cultivate her imagination? Think of the ways in which muscle is developed, by which skill is acquired.

Noise.—What is the relation between a nurse's imagination and the noise that disturbs the sick so seriously. A very close relation indeed! If a nurse had her imagination so trained that she could appreciate how noise jarred on sensitive nerves, would she be more careful, would she try to correct her noisy habits? What are the chief causes of hospital noise in your hospital? Constructive difficulties may have something to do with them. Elevators may be too close to patients. Diet kitchens may be too close to wards. These defects are not for pupil nurses to remedy.

If the question were, "what is the chief cause of noise

due to nurses in hospitals?" it might be clearer. Study carefully your own department for one day and night, and note every kind of noise that disturbs, day noises and night noises, and how they might be prevented. In nine cases out of ten, the chief cause of noise, apart from crying babies, and the noise from delirious or suffering patients, will be found to be the human voice, though not always of nurses. Staff doctors are often heard talking in the corridors in the same tone they would use if going through a factory. Internes are frequent offenders also in this respect. But since nurses are more numerous than either of these other offenders and since they are very directly and constantly concerned with the comfort of the patient, they should be keenly alive to the necessity of maintaining quietness in the sick room. They are alive to the need of quietness when they enter. Instinctively, people in general speak in hushed tones and subdue their movements when they are in the presence of sickness. When does this feeling of the necessity for quietness for the sick leave nurses? Can it be regained? A list of the causes of preventable noises in hospitals would include: Banging of doors, rattling of basins, creaking of hinges, flapping of window-shades, sometimes, noisy handling of chart files, moving of furniture, collecting of trays; the list might be continued indefinitely. These causes should be made a subject for real study by every class.

Can your imagination help you to answer this question? If you were a really ill typhoid fever patient, how would it feel to be placed in a bed near the door of a ward through which doctors, internes, nurses, visitors must pass every few minutes in the day? If your temperature were hovering up around 104°F. would it enliven you and help you to combat the fever by having this constant stream of people on different errands, passing your bed? Would a little more imagination help us to place really ill patients where they would not have to endure this? Would it make us a little more thoughtful?

The husband of a patient who had been in the hospital two weeks, marched into a hospital office one evening with high indignation written on his face. He had come, he said, to make a protest about the way his wife was being treated in the hospital. He was angry clear through, he said. Inquiry revealed that the sole cause of this outburst was that the doctor had said his wife might sit up in bed and the nurse hadn't attended to it. The nurse told his wife that she couldn't find a back-rest. In reality she had made no serious attempt to find one, had not reported to the head nurse that she couldn't find one. She didn't think it made any special difference. She did not imagine how it felt to have been on one's back in bed for two weeks. She did not realize that "sitting up" may be, and often is, a red-letter event in an unusual chapter in a life history. She realized it only after a patient had grown indignant and complained, a husband had become irate, and a general ill-feeling toward the hospital had been created.

A Nurse's Experience as a Patient.—A nurse who was twice a patient in the same hospital writes thus of some of her experiences while a patient: "The surgical treatment I received was excellent, but the nursing left much to be desired. The first night I heard the day nurse telling the night nurse 'No. 13 was a new patient, another nurse, and she was sick of nurses.' I had no sleep at all the first night, as my bed was facing the kitchen door, which was left wide open, with the light streaming directly on my face, and the night nurses constantly resorted thither for audible chatter. The second night I was given chloral, and hoped for some sleep; but the day nurse started my preparation for operation before she went off duty at 9 P.M., and left it for the night nurse to finish when convenient, which seemed to be about 1 A.M. Three enemas during the night at two-hourly intervals did not add to the possibility of sleep. The night nurse used to go from one patient to another with the same syringe without any sterilizing, and thought screens for douching, enemas, etc., quite superfluous."

If the imagination of the nurses on duty had been a little more fully developed, would these discomforts have been created for this nurse? Have the patients now in your care any reason to complain of you in the matters this nurse complains of?

Suggested Subject for Written Work.—Make a list of the causes of noise that you have observed in your department with suggestions for their prevention.

FOR DISCUSSION OR REVIEW

1. Explain the term "tact." How can it be cultivated?
2. How may an untactful nurse train herself to be tactful?
3. Show how the quality of imagination in a nurse may affect the comfort of her patients.
4. Apart from standing orders make a list of rules which nurses should observe in connection with new patients.
5. What attitude should a nurse manifest to a patient's friends?
6. Give some suggestions for a nurse in regard to the

management of visitors, mentioning things to be avoided.

7. From your own observation in the hospital what reason have patients had to complain of their treatment by nurses?

8. Apart from the standing and special orders, what does a nurse owe to a patient?

CHAPTER X

Some Ethical Phases of Night Duty

A nurse's first term of night duty is one of the experiences in her life which lives long in her memory. Years later, she will usually be able to recall the names of some of the patients assigned to her care, her own emotions on the first night on duty, and the little happenings that were a part of her initiation into the realities of night service.

Like many other of her life experiences, this one will not come to her labeled "Important." It will come as an ordinary step in her training, but it means for her more real responsibility than she has had to carry heretofore. It means that her character, her moral nature will be tested more severely than when on day duty. Supervision over her is not so close or so constant as she has been accustomed to. To have the care of a number of sick people entrusted to her, as a night nurse has, is not a small responsibility. What are some of the tests of character she will have to meet?

1. *The comfort of the patients* will be more entirely in her hands than on day duty. This is not alone a test of nursing ability but of character. There are numerous things which she might do to add to their comfort which she may leave undone, and no one in authority will be the wiser. There is nothing in the orders concerning many things which she should do, to be true to her best self. Turning a pillow and shaking it for a

restless patient; a gentle rub of the back or limbs; straightening wrinkles from sheets; bathing face and hands; slipping a small pillow here and there to give support to a part; adjusting a larger pillow till it is really comfortable; moistening parched lips; snipping the edge of a roller bandage on an extremity, thus easing pressure on the wounded part; elevating a wounded limb till it is supported gradually and evenly and is comfortable; supporting the knees and thighs by a pillow; careful adjustment of light and arrangement for proper ventilation; a bit of extra covering as needed—these are suggestions of "comfort" methods which need to be adapted to the individual patient, few if any of which will be included in the orders.

What qualities of a nurse's character will be tested by these opportunities for real genuine service to the sick? How far may she excuse herself for neglecting them? What effect will continued neglect of such opportunities have on a nurse's habits? How will indifference to a patient's comfort, even when combined with rigid adherence to orders, influence her desirability as a nurse?

2. *Her good judgment* will be tested more severely than on day duty. Conditional orders are often given as to whether to give or withhold certain medicines. A patient's condition may seem to be growing more critical. She must decide as to whether she shall report the matter.

A sudden serious change may develop which may make it necessary to call the resident physician or the friends of the patient. She does not want to make herself a nuisance by raising unnecessary alarms, or by making too frequent demands on the night supervisor; she does want to have everything possible done for the patient. In a small hospital there may be no night supervisor.

The day supervisors need their rest. Shall she disturb any one or not? These are tests of the make-up and development of the nurse.

3. *Her powers of observation* will be tested. Serious complications or emergencies may occur which she should have noted and perhaps did not. A dressing may accidentally become displaced, leaving the wound exposed to infection. She should notice it. She may often have to judge of the severity of a symptom of which the patient complains. Many patients are highly emotional and make a fuss out of all proportion to the gravity of their condition. She will be open to the charge of harshness and indifference, if she refuses to believe they are suffering and does not apparently try to relieve them. She may give such patients so much attention, because they are noisy and troublesome, that she neglects some silent sufferer who needs special attention.

Hysteria is a term which nurses often use too freely. Nurses who would not think of transgressing the rule in regard to other diseases that a well-trained nurse does not make or announce a diagnosis, and does not prescribe, outside of simple nursing measures for comfort or relief, nurses who have only a glimmering of understanding of what hysteria is, will glibly announce that this or that patient is suffering from hysteria. They do not know that the ablest physicians are often perplexed and deceived in regard to such cases, and unwilling to venture a positive opinion, while frequently with the recklessness of inexperience and ignorance, a nurse after being one night with a patient, will freely pass judgment and announce that her patient has hysteria. Even if it be true, it is never wise for a nurse to announce it. Few things will give greater offense to the patient or his family than such an announcement, and when it has to be made, it should come from the doctor in charge of the case, and not the nurse.

It is no part of a nurse's business to diagnose disease, yet every day one may find nurses doing it. Guesses in many cases will necessarily be made. The patient will often announce his own diagnosis of his case, but every nurse should study to avoid expressing her opinions as to the disease a patient is suffering from. To do so shows a lack of training, a lack of that fine sense of propriety which nurses should try to possess.

This rule holds just as good in regard to the ailments of nurses as in regard to patients. A nurse in announcing that her roommate or next door neighbor in the nurses' home is ill, adds perhaps the statement, "Her throat is dreadfully sore. I think she has diphtheria," and the story grows, as it is passed around. Some nurses seem to feel that if a *nurse* is ill they may freely express their own opinions as to the disease, even if a doctor has not examined her, or if he is withholding a diagnosis till he feels more certain.

Think over some of the bad results which may follow a nurse going out of her province and announcing her diagnosis of an illness. What results may such a habit lead to in a hospital, in a nurse's home, also when engaged as a private nurse?

4. There will come to a night nurse the temptation to spend too much time with a patient who is congenial to her and to neglect others less congenial. This temptation is not peculiar to night duty, but with less close supervision of her methods the night nurse is the more likely to yield to it.

5. *Attire.*—A night nurse on special duty is frequently tempted to be careless in regard to the attire in which she appears in corridors, before doctors, internes, and

orderlies. Make a note of the things to be avoided in this respect.

6. *Loyalty to the institution* and its rules will be tested in various ways while on night duty. She will often find it inconvenient to enforce rules regarding hours when visitors must leave, and lights must be out; she will perhaps be tempted to gossip with internes and doctors and to forget the proper limitations placed on duty in regard to professional relations with men, of whatever class. She may easily become the subject of unpleasant gossip by some indiscretion of this kind, which is usually noted by some patient or fellow-worker.

Is a night nurse on duty at liberty to provide lunches for internes who happen to make late rounds, using the food supplies provided for her, or for the use of patients, for that purpose? What bad results are liable to follow if a nurse begins this practice?

7. *Her Honesty will be Tested.*—Much may be done that should not be done and the matter covered up.

She may be tempted to absent herself from her ward or department for some time, leaving no one in her place. She may neglect to make rounds as frequently as ordered to make sure that all is well.

She may permit herself to fall asleep while on duty and neglect to carry out certain orders, or neglect her patients.

She may try to cover up her failures by making false entries on her records.

She may wilfully waste hospital money by allowing unnecessary lights to burn, and this is a form of untrustworthiness.

She may neglect to "own up" to the head nurse or principal of the school that certain things occurred or were not attended to. The nurse who "owns up" is the nurse who inspires confidence. She shows she has that fine sense of honor so essential in a good nurse. It is not always an easy thing to do. It requires courage. Sometimes the warring impulses in a nurse's heart will suggest to her "why say anything about it? It probably will never be known; why bother about a little matter that is not important?" Every nurse knows by experience this war with one's own conscience. How she meets these apparently simple and unimportant tests is a matter that is going to count tremendously in the moral influence she exerts on others, on the moral atmosphere of the school, and these tests leave their own indelible mark on her personal character.

Principles are inconvenient things, sometimes. Matters of expediency suggest one course; duty and conscience, another, but there is no question as to the ultimate reward of putting what is right before the thing which at the time seems more convenient, expedient, or to be preferred.

8. *Accuracy* is closely related to truthfulness. It is an important quality for a nurse to cultivate, and night duty is an especially good time for her to put forth special effort to develop this quality. It is her business to be able to state facts accurately, definitely, in regard to every patient under her care. Under average conditions, a nurse will have some patients sleeping most of the night; others who are restless and easily disturbed; others who are unable to sleep because of pain or discomfort. Her reports should never consist of vague generalities such as "slept pretty well" or "had a good night." A patient who did not bother the nurse very much or make many demands on her may easily be said to have "had a good night," when in reality the night nurse did not know whether he slept at all, or

how much. Her reports should state definitely the approximate number of hours each patient slept, except, perhaps, those who are convalescent and whose general condition needs no special watching at night. A patient's record may state that he "slept pretty well," while he complains that he got little or no sleep at all. Quite often a patient who lies awake for an hour or two (the night hours often seem to be more than sixty minutes in length) will complain that he was awake all night. The nurse should visit each patient often enough to know how many hours, approximately, he slept or was awake.

What is true of accuracy as it relates to sleep is just as true in other details. An inaccurate nurse guesses about much which she should know and be able to speak definitely and positively. She often carries her guesses into the realm of medicines and does not bother to measure drugs of various kinds. She records guesses as exact facts.

A night nurse was seen pouring whiskey into an ordinary drinking glass. "How much whiskey is the patient supposed to have that you are preparing that dose for?" she was asked by the night supervisor who was passing. "A half ounce" was the nurse's reply. "You have nearer two ounces than a half ounce in that glass," the supervisor replied. The nurse argued that she knew a half ounce without measuring it. On measuring the dose which the nurse had poured out, it was found that she was giving the patient an ounce and a half of whiskey instead of a half ounce. She had been carefully taught to measure drugs, but she did not class whiskey as a drug. She did not do as she was taught. She thought it did not make any difference if he did get a little more than was ordered. She was willing to guess and take chances instead of giving medicines as she had been taught. Especially she was given to guessing on night duty when she thought it would not be noticed. She was reporting on her records that the patient had been given a half-ounce dose of whiskey when in reality he had been given three times that amount. What moral principle did she violate?

Apart from the moral principle involved in this transaction, what bad effects might accrue to patients as a result of this kind of ethical failure in a nurse?

System.—While on day duty a first year nurse's work is largely planned for her by head nurses, or by nurses with more experience. On night duty she has the planning of the details of her work herself to a great extent. The comfort of the patients will be influenced to a considerable extent by her systematic habits or the lack of them.

It is usual to try to have the wards quiet and lights shaded or turned out by nine o'clock so that sick people can settle down to sleep. Most duties which would interfere with the patient's sleeping will probably be attended to before that time. Patients who are likely to need constant watchfulness and attention will have screens adjusted; night lights will be in readiness. Causes of noise will be studied and measures taken to prevent. The nurse herself will wear soft-soled shoes and cultivate gentle footsteps and movements.

The orders will be studied and plans made for carrying out the duties with quietness and "despatch." Basins, glasses, and appliances will be cleaned up as she goes along, and not allowed to accumulate and add to the morning work. She will be told the earliest hour when morning temperatures should be taken, and will be careful not to wake patients at unnecessarily early hours to carry out a routine duty. She will try to study how to systematize her work so that she gets through without being "rushed" in the last half hour. All the time she is arranging her work she will be developing that quality called "Executive Ability," which is so much in demand.

Ten nurses can follow orders, can do routine work well, if planned and directed by someone else, where one will be found who has developed the qualities of planning for others, of getting work done without needless fuss and friction. It is the one nurse who has cultivated this quality before and during training who finds positions seeking her; she is in demand. Her services are worth more than those of the other ten who have not this quality.

The Nurse's Health.—The turning of night into day, of working hours into sleeping hours, is never or rarely accomplished without some difficulty in regard to sleep and general health. The general experience of night duty is that it causes physical depression in a greater or less degree. For this reason a nurse needs to guard her health even more carefully than when on day duty. Out-of-door recreation, taken some time during the hours of sunshine, is imperative if general vitality is to be kept up to the ordinary mark. Sunshine is a great vitalizer and restorer. There is a wonderful power in "God's out-of-doors" to minister to our minds which exercise their subtle influence over our bodies; to increase our power to resist disease and the depressing influence of the sick room; to quiet irritated nerves, to keep us sweet tempered and at our best.

The temptation to violate the rule which requires night nurses to be in bed between certain hours of the day comes to most nurses, yet both she and the patients suffer if a nurse fails to get the sleep required. It takes a few days to get accustomed to sleeping during the daytime. If a nurse is unable to sleep after she has used all the measures she knows of to procure sleep, the matter should be reported to the principal of the school.

Experience teaches much in regard to this matter. Perhaps a nurse is indulging in strong tea or coffee just before retiring; perhaps the room she sleeps in is not well ventilated or darkened; perhaps there are house noises, noise made by other nurses, which the principal could quietly and promptly check if she knew of their occurrence. In any case, since a nurse cannot do her best work without a reasonable amount of sleep, it is important that everything possible be done to help her secure it.

The Avoidance of Friction.—The dividing line between a day nurse's responsibility and that which properly belongs to night nurses is not always as clearly drawn as we might desire. There are numerous opportunities for friction and unpleasantness, which may react unfavorably on the patients. Such friction often renders nurses unhappy, and the cause is usually so trivial that one grows impatient with nurses who yield to it.

Let it be understood clearly that since nurses are in training and forming habits, it is no real kindness in a nurse to cover up laxity or neglect in some other nurse who is being trained. Training should be helping *every* nurse to overcome such habits, and by covering up the results of careless habits we help a nurse to become more careless.

The manner in which acts of neglect or carelessness are brought to a nurse's attention has much to do with the way she accepts reproof or reminder. If the lapse is apparently accidental we can overlook it in a nurse who is usually careful. If it seems to occur so often as to be habitual with her it has a different aspect. Motive and habit need to be considered.

A badly soiled basin was found one morning by the day nurse in charge of the corridor. She called the night nurse's attention to it. The night nurse declared it was there when she went on duty, that she had not touched the basin but had left it where she found it. The next morning the night nurse's attention was again called to the basin; it had been carefully left for her to clean up. She refused; sharp words followed. Other nurses were called in to bear witness in the case. The tempest grew. Much ill-feeling was created. Finally, each nurse determined to carry the matter of her innocence to the principal. They came, unhappy, crying and angry, with their stories. Two or three days had elapsed. What course should the principal have pursued in the matter? How might such unhappiness have been prevented by each nurse? Was the cause of the difficulty enough to have caused the nurses such unhappiness? After the unhappiness and trouble caused by the incident, what should the nurses involved do to minimize the bad effects of the quarrel?

Suggested Subject for Written Work.—Prepare a list of ten suggestions which you would give to a young nurse about to begin her first term of night duty, things to do, things to avoid.

FOR DISCUSSION OR REVIEW

1. Mention at least a dozen "comfort methods" which a night nurse may use, which are not likely to be in the standing orders.

2. State why or how a nurse's character is likely to be more severely tested on night duty than on day duty.

3. What effect will continued neglect of small things, by which she might add to a patient's comfort, have on her own character and the general quality of the service she renders?

4. Give reasons why nurses should be careful not to announce that a certain patient has hysteria.

5. Is the temptation for a nurse to administer sedatives or sleep-producing drugs to noisy or troublesome patients, without orders, one that is likely to present itself to night nurses especially? State your own observations on this point. In case a nurse yields to this temptation, what should be the policy of the principal of the school toward her?

6. If a night nurse discovers that another night nurse is administering sedative drugs without orders, what course should she pursue? Has she any responsibility in the matter?

7. What points should a nurse on special duty at night be careful to observe in regard to her attire?

8. Mention some of the special problems that present themselves to night nurses.

9. At what hour in the morning should a nurse begin to wake patients for temperature taking and the morning work?

10. What suggestions would you give a nurse in managing her morning work?

11. Show how night nurses have special opportunities for developing systematic habits.

12. Outline some important rules of hygiene which night nurses should be careful to observe.

CHAPTER XI

Ethics and the Everyday Routine

Nothing so tests character as the daily routine. We may be able to rise to sublime heights of courage and resourcefulness in times of emergency, and yet easily fail to show the patience, tolerance, faithfulness and good judgment needed in the everyday routine of the ward or department. Here ethical principles have to be weighed quickly and acted on, or the opportunity is gone. Habits assert themselves. The record which we are making every day as practical workers and as high- or low-principled women will probably count for or against us years hence. It may be a hindrance or a help in getting some greatly desired position. This truth is one which nurses should never forget, for probably no class of workers is more dependent on recommendations than are nurses. There is a close relation between recommendations and the daily record of conduct and deportment which a nurse leaves in the hospital.

Permanent Records.—In the efficiency records of a well-organized school there will be found, concerning every nurse, her grade on such points as the following:

Personality { disposition.
neatness.

Quality of work.
Agreeableness to patients.
Conscientiousness in details.
Obedience.
Power of observation.
Reliability.

Systematic habits.
Executive ability.
Health.
Nursing instinct.

The nurse makes these records, the principal keeps them for future reference, when inquiry comes to the hospital in regard to her.

Disposition.—The nurse's general disposition manifested in a thousand ways carries tremendous weight when fitness for different positions has to be considered. A recommendation which states that "Miss Blank is a capable nurse, but—" is not a very desirable recommendation, yet it is the only kind which many principals can conscientiously give to some nurses. It means often that the nurse knows how to nurse, that her technical ability is creditable, but that in disposition or general conduct as a woman there is doubt as to her desirability. A nurse may be a success considered from the standpoint of technic, and a brilliant failure from the standpoint of ethics. The great majority of failures on the part of nurses to measure up to the reasonable expectations of the public are failures in disposition or conduct; *they are ethical failures.*

Is a nurse inclined to be sullen or sulky under reproof? It becomes a part of her record if she is.

Does she give way to anger easily?

Has she the quiet dignity of manner so desirable in a nurse?

Is she inclined to make confidential friends of her patients on very brief acquaintance?

Is she careful in her habits of speech?

Is she addicted to slang, or does she indulge in vulgar expletives and coarse jests?

Is she always alert to observe the niceties of conduct in her relation to her patients?

Is she faithful in small details?

Is she inclined to criticize the management?

Does she openly discuss the methods and failings of physicians?

Is she careful in all her dealings with men—doctors, patients, orderlies, patients' friends, other men—or is her conduct such that she becomes a subject for gossip or criticism because of indiscretion in this respect?

Is she a chronic grumbler?

Does she act as if she were a much-maligned mortal, whose misfortunes were always due to someone else?

Does she cherish the foolish notion that someone in authority has a secret grudge against her and that she can never expect to be dealt with justly?

Is she able to get along sweetly with her associates, or are there liable to be signs of friction wherever she happens to be on duty?

Is she afraid of doing too much for her patients? Does she carry with her the spirit of glad, willing service? Is her spirit selfish or unselfish?

Is she careful to observe rules, or does she need constant watching?

Is she earnest in her desire and efforts to improve and to correct her own faults of disposition or habit?

Improvement.—These are some of the points at which every nurse is being tested in the everyday routine. Perfection is not expected of her. Improvement is rightly expected. Training should be improving her. It is the nurse who, after having her attention repeatedly called to the need of improvement in some particular yet shows no sign of improvement, no effort to correct the fault or weakness, who is the big problem in many a school. Her technical work may be good, her disposition most deplorable. She may be tolerated and allowed to finish her course, because she commits no open or flagrant misdemeanor that has been discovered, that seems to justify her dismissal; but how can a nurse who has proven an ethical failure hope for her training school to recommend her for positions where she will have an opportunity to set an example of unethical conduct and unworthy disposition to others?

During the first year, before habits are too firmly fixed, there is excellent opportunity for any nurse who earnestly desires it to "mend her ways," to reform her habits, and to constantly endeavor to live up to the personal ideal she should keep before her. Her ideal should change as she sees a little deeper into the meaning and end of life and of nursing, but it should never descend to a lower plane.

The Need of Solitude.—Every individual needs her seasons of solitude when, apart from the distractions of life and away from the influence of other minds, she can look into her own soul, take a square look at the record she is making, and see as in a mirror the points where effort at readjustment, at strengthening weak places in character, should be made. This time of solitude a nurse will rarely get unless she insists on it. Much time is wasted by nurses in off-duty hours by aimless gossiping about the incidents of the day, gossip which may be harmful to the nurse, even if not malicious, because of the habit of gossip which she is forming.

Quality of Work.—How is the quality of work estimated? Chiefly in regard to thoroughness; partly in relation to what has been taught; partly in relation to improvement in regard to details; partly by the spirit which pervades the work. Is a nurse thoughtful in seeing little things to be done for the comfort of the patients, or the reverse? Does her work have that finished appearance that is so desirable? Is she neat in her personal habits? Is she in the habit of tidying up as she goes along, or does she leave a trail of soiled basins, glasses, dishes, appliances, which she means to put in order "when she gets around to them?" Just a few such nurses who never learn to put things in order as they go along may easily make for a hospital the undesirable reputation of lack of neatness and cleanliness.

The reputation of the hospital rests more on the quality of its nursing than on any other single thing connected with its management. Good nursing consists in attention to small details, and the nurses are adding to, or marring, the good reputation of the hospital every day of their lives.

One of the common failings of pupil nurses is to neglect answering a call from one patient because they happen to be busy with another. There are perhaps few things more frequently complained of in regard to hospitals than the neglect to answer calls promptly. Nurses in general are altogether too prone to excuse themselves on plea of being "busy." It is an important part of a nurse's training to develop the ability to attend properly to the wants of several patients and keep them all happy and satisfied, with no reasonable ground for feeling neglected. A nurse in a very short time should be able to show that she can be busy with one patient and not neglect another for whom she is equally responsible. This calls for system, and even more for the manifestation of the spirit of cheerful readiness to do, which is quickly felt by patients and helps immensely in making them more willing to wait. A nurse who tries and succeeds in making her patients happy, and inspiring them with the feeling that she has a real solicitude for their comfort, has done much for the reputation of the hospital so far as her patients and his friends are concerned.

The old time-worn complaint of the patient who signalled for half an hour for a nurse to bring him a drink of water and then had to go without it is based on a foundation of fact in most hospitals. Even as small a thing as that helps to mar the reputation of the hospital so far as its nursing is concerned.

Would you consider a nurse a success who was able to satisfy one patient, when she could give him her whole attention, but a failure in attending satisfactorily to the wants of three or four? How may a nurse develop the ability to so plan her work, and so manage herself, that she can keep several patients comfortable and well cared for with no reasonable ground for feeling neglected?

Powers of Observation.—A nurse's efficiency is judged to a large degree by the extent to which she cultivates her power of observation and uses it in the daily routine. A physician states that "the whole science of medicine rests on the power of observation. The modern conception that many diseases are due to micro-organisms we owe to this quality being born in men like Pollender, Davaine, Pasteur and Koch."

It is so easy to get into ruts in making records—noting only the routine things and failing to notice various important matters concerning patients that are readily seen when pointed out—that many nurses follow the course of least resistance. If Florence Nightingale had done this the world today would practically have forgotten that she lived. It was that quality of keenness, that insistent habit of note-taking regarding the care of the sick that helped her to lay the foundation for nursing education as we have it today. If she had waited, as so many nurses do, to have every bit of knowledge duly administered by some one appointed for the purpose, if she had failed to see things all around her which bore on the thing she was anxious to learn, she could never have accomplished the work she did. It should be the ambition of every pupil to gather up scattered bits of nursing knowledge and to cultivate to the fullest extent her observing powers concerning her patients and her work. The nurse who has this quality of keenness well developed has usually a fine enthusiasm regarding her work and is likely to find positions waiting for her when she is ready to leave the school.

The Nursing Instinct.—What is it? Is it that acute perception of the importance of small things in the comfort of a patient—that sense that prompts a nurse to see a hundred small things that would make him more comfortable and do them, while another nurse contents herself with doing what she considers important, and sees nothing further which she might have done?

If a nurse seems to be lacking in nursing instinct, can it be cultivated during training? If so, how?

Professional versus Confidential Relations.—From the entrance of a nurse to the training school, she hears that her relations with patients must be "strictly professional," and she well knows the necessity of this rule. Yet there are nurses, many of them, who never seem to be able to keep their relations with patients within professional limits. They have a "confiding" way with them, and in spite of positive prohibitions will, before they have known their patients twenty-four hours, be found relating to them their own private affairs which, certainly, sick people should not be bothered with. Even "love affairs" are often unfolded to patients on a few hours' acquaintance.

A bright, attractive, young woman was deserted by her husband and left with two children to be cared for. The children were placed with relatives, and through the influence of friends she was admitted to a training school. On entrance she was admonished privately and positively that her disappointment in marriage must not be made known to patients, neither were her children to be discussed with them. In spite of repeated admonitions, in spite of all that anyone could do, she continued to tell patients of her disappointment, of the needs of her children for whom she had to provide clothing, until in justice to the reputation of the school and to the other nurses she had to be dismissed. Patients were sorry for her and gave her gifts of money for her children, and the discipline of the school in this respect was made exceedingly difficult while she remained. Knowing the necessity she was under to become able to earn a living for herself and her children, it was hard to say to her that she could not continue in training, but whose fault was it that it had to be done?

She had many other good qualities—was unselfish, faithful to the needs of her patients, quick to grasp the technical part of her training. Should her good qualities have enabled her to complete her course, in spite of this serious failing? How was this failing likely to affect the other nurses and the school generally?

A nurse who was exceptionally capable along technical lines had the habit of establishing confidential or semi-confidential relations with men patients in particular, especially private-room patients, but frequently with ward patients. It became known that she was in the habit of receiving letters from many of the men she nursed, after they had left the hospital. Quite often the correspondence died out in a few weeks or months, through its intensity, but new correspondents took the place of those who dropped out, and the habit became a standing joke among other nurses. Also, it became a problem to know where to place her on duty. In the women's departments or women's wards she proved most capable. In the men's wards she was inclined to be "confiding" and familiar in her manner in dealing with men in general, yet nothing of a really scandalous nature was discovered. Should such a nurse have been allowed to graduate? Is the failure to maintain strictly professional relations with men sufficient to justify dismissal? How many nurses do you know personally who have failed in this respect?

Suggested Subject for Written Work.—In what ways may a nurse's disposition interfere with her success as a nurse? Mention some methods which a nurse may use to correct faults in her own disposition.

FOR DISCUSSION OR REVIEW

1. Make a list of the points in a nurse's history in the school which should become part of the permanent records.
2. How is the quality of a nurse's work estimated?
3. Show how the quality of a nurse's work affects the reputation of the hospital and its standing with the public.
4. When a nurse is in charge of several private patients, mention some points which she should be careful to observe in order that none may feel neglected.
5. Give reasons why a nurse should not discuss her private affairs with patients.
6. What do you understand by the term "professional relations?"

7. If a nurse is given to having favorites among her patients, giving special attention to one and "visiting" with him while neglecting others, how should she be dealt with?

8. Show how the vice of favoritism may affect the happiness and welfare of patients and the reputation of the hospital.

9. What do you understand by the phrase "nursing instinct?"

SECTION II

CHAPTER XII

The Cost of Training

Apart from the natural blessings which we enjoy—fresh air, sun, rain, etc., few things in this world that are worth having are secured without some one paying the cost. Yet it is one of the commonest human failings to take for granted much of great value that comes to us, and to unconsciously but utterly fail in appreciating, at anything like their real cost, many of the blessings that we receive.

Not many children are able to appreciate until many years of life have passed, the cost in dollars and cents of their maintenance and education—apart entirely from other aspects of their life which cannot be reckoned in terms of money.

Few college students who do not pay their own way through college are able to estimate, at anything like its real value, the cost of their education. Few nurses take time to consider that the board, room, heat, light, instruction and supervision and all the other things which come to them while in training have all to be paid for by somebody. None of these things are to be had without cost.

At different times the suggestion has been made that nurses should pay for their tuition, and be able to exercise more choice in regard to the various details of their training than is now the rule. But serious attention has seldom been given to the matter of such cost to the nurse, should such a change be made, nor to the fact that many of the best nurses now in the field would have been barred from being nurses, had they been required to have sufficient capital to pay in money for their training.

The cost of a year in college for a young woman varies from about $300 to $1000 a year and upward. A Wellesley graduate of 1915 states that the general cost in that college of room, board and tuition is $500 a year. This is exclusive of books, laboratory fees, and various other incidental but necessary expenses, and takes no account of clothing, the cost of which depends on the young woman herself. The young woman who gave this information secured soon after her graduation a position as welfare secretary at $75 a month, out of which must be paid the cost of her room, board, laundry, etc. Estimate what a four years' college course costs a young woman at the rate quoted above, including probable expenses for books, clothing, laboratory fees and other incidental expenses including, also, traveling expenses, if she lived three hundred miles from the college.

What advantages or disadvantages does she have as compared with a nurse graduating from a hospital, from the standpoint of a woman worker?

Compare her opportunities with the opportunities of the graduate nurse as to service to humanity, and possible financial reward for her labors.

The cost of a nurse's training is not easily estimated, and many hospitals do not attempt to keep the cost of the training school separate from general administration expenses. As is the case with colleges, the cost varies greatly in different localities and in different hospitals in the same locality. In some hospitals a monthly money allowance is paid to pupil nurses. In others, books, uniforms, etc., are provided, but no allowance. All such items enter into the cost of the maintenance of a pupil nurse. The number of paid nurse supervisors is determined by each institution, and this number may vary from one to fifty or more. In estimating the cost of head nurses and supervisors, apart from their salaries, must be reckoned the items of their housing accommodation, board, laundry, books and materials for teaching, care in sickness, and other incidental expenses. The cost of the supervisor's room or suite in an average hospital would range from $10 to $40 or $50 a month, or more depending on the number of rooms, their furnishings and the various items and privileges which go with the room, and which a worker living in an ordinary apartment house would have to pay for. Calculate the annual cost of a suite of rooms consisting of a sitting room, bedroom, and private bath which is heated, furnished, and lighted, if such were in an apartment house or family hotel.

Throughout the United States and Canada, millions of dollars are invested in training school buildings or homes for nurses, and large sums of money are expended every year in the heating, lighting, furnishing and general maintenance and management of those homes. In estimating the cost of training nurses all these expenses must be included, and the amount of capital invested in such buildings should not be left out of consideration.

For purposes of illustration the cost of supporting a pupil nurse has been secured from several representative hospitals in different cities and different parts of the country.

In Memorial Hospital, Worcester, Mass., the cost of maintaining a pupil nurse is stated to be slightly over $1.00 per day for the whole term of training—somewhat over $1000 for each pupil for a three years' course. This includes room, board, laundry, tuition, supervision, care in sickness, etc.

In New York Hospital, New York City, the cost of maintaining and training a nurse is $1.58 per day, excluding the rent of two buildings which are used exclusively in the housing of nurses. This item should be charged against the training school and increases the cost to $1.71 per day or over $600 a year—more than the cost in many colleges. The items of expense furnished by the New York Hospital are as follows:

Salaries, directress of nurses, assistants, pupil nurses and instructors and a physician	$8,008
Salaries, domestics	2,646
Books	22
Insurance on building	414
Laundry	2,112
Heat, light, and power	5,785
Gas	568
Repairs, etc.	375
Kitchen	990
Food	21,148
Administration	1,800
Commencement expenses	700
Drugs, medicines, etc.	300
Bedding, household supplies, etc.	1,860
Rent	5,800
Total	$62,528

The expense items furnished by the Massachussetts General Hospital are given approximately as follows, covering a nurse's three years' course:

Uniforms, books, stationery, etc.	$70.21
Board	1170.00
Laundry	113.67
Proportion of salaries, wages and board of training school officers and employees	265.00
Insurance, depreciation, interest on investment, electricity, gas, etc., on nurse's home	505.80
Total	$2124.68

Miss Anna C. Jamme, Director, Bureau of Registration of Nurses, California, estimates the cost of training a pupil nurse for three years at $1512. Room and board are estimated at $25 per month, total $900. Laundry averages $9 per month, total $324. The balance being allotted to allowance with tuition or instruction considered free.

Attention may be called to the thought that the special nursing of private patients done by pupil nurses in many hospitals, reimburses the hospital in part at least, for the expense of maintenance, and to a degree, this holds true. Yet on the other hand, the pupil, while on special duty, is being taught, and is gaining experience which is of great value to her when she goes out as an independent worker. Many students are glad to pay for the opportunity to do "real work" that will afford some practical experience with everyday responsibilities, that will help to give the confidence in one's powers needed for effective work, and that will add to the chances for securing the kind of work desired. The cost of training has many angles which should be discussed, but one point to be emphasized is that a hospital training school offers advantages over almost all other schools, for a nurse with ambition and without capital, to secure an education that will fit her at once on graduation to earn an independent livelihood. It fits her for a vocation that affords unusual opportunities for advancement and for satisfying service to humanity.

Other Aspects of the Cost of Training.—The cost of an education cannot always be reckoned in terms of money. Not infrequently a student enters college with high purposes and the noblest ideals of life, and leaves it with his ideals gone, his life purpose thrown to the winds, his character seared, his influence changed from good to bad. Many never recover the ground lost. What influences are responsible for this change? Mention some ways by which it might come to pass? To what extent is a student responsible for this retrograde condition?

A nurse *may* pay the cost of training in lost ideals, in changed purposes, in impaired character and influence, but she does not need to. It is rare, if ever, that an individual is placed in a position in which he cannot do right, and live right, if he is determined to do so.

A Fundamental Ethical Principle.—Analyze the following statement of ethical principles showing whether the writer is wrong or right in affirming what he believes to be a fundamental truth.

"The center of character is found in the will to do right, and it cannot be too much emphasized that where it is present, other lacks may be excused; and where it is absent nothing else can take its place. The will to do right is also possible to every one, and in all circumstances. With it every one can make a beginning and all may meet on the plane of a common faithfulness. The ignorant, the poor, the savage, may be faithful to their ideal of right and thereby win the approval of all moral beings. This does not imply their perfection in any sense, but only a right attitude of will toward righteousness. This furnishes the indispensable condition of all moral development. So much is possible to every one; less than this can be accepted from none."*

Some writer has said that "It is good to have money and the things tha tmoney can buy; but it's good, too, to check up once in awhile, and make sure you haven't lost the thing that money can't buy." This bit of wisdom might be slightly changed in its wording and

* Principles of Ethics. Bowne.

applied to nurses and a nursing education. There is a danger of losing something out of our lives and out of nursing that we cannot afford to lose or to value lightly.

Dangers which Beset.—In an address to pupil nurses* Dr. Richard Cabot calls attention to three great dangers which beset nurses.

1. Callousness, or the routine spirit.
2. Narrowness.
3. Dissipation of energy.

Discussing the subject of callousness or the routine spirit, Dr. Cabot expresses himself thus: "Our profession, the profession to which you as nurses and we as physicians contribute what we can, brings us constantly into the closest contact with human souls. We are with our fellow-creatures in their hours of storm and stress when what is deepest and truest in them comes to light. Such contact is sure to affect us in one of two ways. It can ennoble us or it can make us callous. There is no other alternative. Familiarity with the great spiritual experiences that attend birth, death, and bereavement, with the awful perplexity of choosing between one life and another, and the awful desolation of the sufferer who learns for the first time his malady is incurable, drives us all either to shut our ears to the poignant message of our work, hopeless of understanding its meaning, or else opens every sense and every faculty to meet the world's revelations, with a faith that is the essence of religion."

Continuing, Dr. Cabot says: "I have watched nurses become coarsened, hardened by their work. It is inevitable when nursing is only a means of winning a livelihood. You cannot pass through such an ordeal without showing the scars. We must pass through a fire that consumes if it does not purify. A man can deal with leather

* Massachussetts General Hospital.

or with hemp and be but little changed by it; but he cannot deal with human suffering, terror, and temptation, with the desperate struggle of the fallen to get upon his feet again, and utter despair of passionate love confronted with vacancy, without being forced to meet, and as best he can, answer the great problems of human life and destiny. By a well-known process all but the finest types of prison chaplain soon begin to show the deadening effect of meeting familiarly the great and sacred crises of human life over and over again until they become commonplace. Unconsciously and inevitably we are all of us infected with the same smug and business-like view of death, sin and suffering, unless the spirit of religion defends us.

"*Our Profession Cannot Remain Secular.*—If it attempts to do so, it becomes a trade and a low one. What do I mean by the spirit of religion in the work of nurse or physician? I mean the missionary, not the proselyting spirit, but the spirit of service, the sense of working for a cause that is absolutely and infinitely worth while, in which we can spend ourselves without stint, without restraint, without reserve. The Greek doctrine of the golden mean, of moderation in all things, is the full opposite of the spirit of religion as I understand it. It is impossible for the world to get, or for us to give, too much of the kind of service I am speaking of. It is its own reward, and the more of it you give, the richer you become. Absolute loyalty to the world's needs, wherever found, is the sum and substance of it all. Wherever there is the greatest need of me, there is my home, and paradise can offer no greater blessing. It is the soldier's creed; it is the creed of the devotee, the world over, and it must be our creed if we are to face the facts, the plain everyday facts of our work. Most of us don't face them. Most of our training has the effect of blinding and deafening us to one-half (and that the most vital half) of the facts before us. To concentrate attention day in and day out on physical processes, without any attempt to go deeper into their meaning, or into the life of the being to whom they belong, is to kill out our sensitiveness to the other manifestations of that life.

"We deal with human life, not with human bodies alone, and yet we are trained exclusively in the care of bodies. No wonder that the souls in those bodies rebel, now and then, and demand someone who recognizes their existence; or else, what is worse, catch from the nurse the materialistic and mechanical view of things toward which all the nurse's training tends. When our training schools admit that to minister to a human being we must know the whole thing, and not only half of him, then it will be impossible any longer to keep them secular, and the spirit of religion will bring about a reorganization of the training there given, and of the type of nurse that graduates. Such nurses will prove the following:

1. "The religious spirit is one that can't be discouraged, for there's no uncertainty about our venture as we see it. The road may turn either way, to life or to death; in any case it must be full of opportunity that we want, the opportunity for service, for sacrifice, for courage and cheerfulness under strain, for education and experience, and for knitting closer the bonds of friendship with all sorts and conditions of men.

2. "The religious spirit is one that can't be hurt, shocked or wounded. It is invulnerable to insult, taunt, annoyance—so small, so puny they seem, as we look through and behind them to the prize of our high calling.

3. "Failure does not seem to touch the religious man,

for to fail in the ordinary sense is to be taught the weak point in his armor, what he needed most to discover, and so to strengthen.

4. "Such a person is like a united army, his powers all dominated by a single motive, his eye single. This gives the great calm, the deep, all-pervasive happiness which shines in such people's faces. We all know such and marvel at it.

5. "Such a person can't but be enthusiastic, because he is always finding what is surprising and fresh; fresh meaning, fresh value in the old, fresh opportunity and experience in the new.

6. "Such a person is everybody's friend because he finds everybody interesting.

"With this spirit in our work we cannot help seeing and fighting against the dangers that beset our profession."

Suggested Subject for Written Work.—What is mechanical service? How may a nurse guard against mechanical service while in training?

QUESTIONS FOR DISCUSSION OR REVIEW

1. What do you regard as the center of character?
2. Show how one's attitude of mind and ideals of right conduct may influence such duties as, giving medicines, giving baths, keeping records, taking temperatures.
3. What is faith? Show how a steady firm faith in the Infinite is necessary for a nurse's peace of mind and how it helps her to become a better nurse.
4. What is callousness in nursing? What daily preventive measures would you recommend a nurse to use?
5. To what extent is a nurse in training responsible for losing her highest ideals of life? To what extent is she the product of her environment?

6. Are we ever placed in situations where it is impossible to do right, if we honestly want to do right? Give illustrations to prove that this is, or is not, so.

7. What general measures may one use to help her to retain interest in the things of eternal value, while in the pressure of daily studies and duties in a training school?

8. Show how a nurse may maintain a proper interest in the spiritual side of her patient's nature, and be entirely free from "the proselyting spirit" which is mentioned in the quotation from Dr. Cabot.

9. What is the missionary spirit which Dr. Cabot insists is essential to the highest type of nurse?

CHAPTER XIII

Good Tone in the Training School

What is meant by "tone" in a school is, briefly, the general or prevailing character of the school as it relates to morals, manners, or sentiment. It should be remembered that the spirit and tone of the school has a tremendous influence on the general reputation of the hospital in any community. It is reflected by the nurses in a thousand ways every day. One who is accustomed to hospitals can, even in a brief tour through a hospital, determine to some degree the prevailing tone of the school.

Two Types of Schools.—In one hospital, one notices nurses neatly attired going about their work with a serious quiet demeanor. Professional courtesies are exchanged with doctors in a dignified way as they come and go. Patients' calls are responded to quickly and quietly. Doors are opened and closed noiselessly. No chattering is heard in corridors. There is an air of alertness and consideration for the patients' needs, and of quiet dignity about the place that gives a feeling of confidence in the general management, and in the personnel of the nursing staff.

In another hospital, one notes the absence of these things. Nurses and doctors greet each other with a boisterous "Hullo." In one place, one even notices a doctor standing with his hand on a nurse's shoulder as she sits at the chart table. One hears nurses calling to each other in corridors, and notes that they fail to use the title "Miss" frequently as they address each other. A Miss Shepherd is given the nickname "Sheppy," Miss Jackson is "Jackie." Others have similar distinguishing titles—nicknames used without malice, no doubt, but showing the lack of that sense of propriety which is so desirable. As one goes through the corridor, one sees a nurse catheterizing a patient in a ward of four beds without screens, and in full view of the corridor. Flippant remarks about patients are overheard. Nurses and internes laugh and joke with each other as they meet, and act as if they never have heard the rule that, "Conversations with doctors and internes while on duty must be limited to professional matters." There is a free and easy air about the place that is the result of lack of training, lack of discipline, lack of a proper conception of what hospital etiquette is, or what a hospital atmosphere should be. From which school would a well-bred refined nurse prefer to graduate?

The Individual Nurse's Responsibility.—It has been stated before, and is repeated for the sake of emphasis, that from the day a probationer arrives in a school she is helping to create the moral atmosphere in which she and other nurses are to live. The hospital and the training school will be either better or worse because she has been a member of the training school family. She does not come to the school as a blank sheet of paper to receive impressions She brings with her, her own personality, her own standards, her own habits. She contributes something to the moral atmosphere of the school every day she is in it. It is for each individual nurse to decide whether she will hold fast to those things which are highest and best and most enduring, whether she will add to the spirit of reverence, of truth, of faith, of courage, of tenderness, that she brought with her to the school—whether these shall be the predominating habits in her nursing life, and whether her influence will help or hinder the formation of right habits in those with whom she associates.

It may be asked, "What can one nurse do to improve conditions such as exist in the latter of the two training schools mentioned?" There are certain to be differences of opinion as to this question, but it is worth thinking over, and worth discussing in class. It will hardly be questioned that a nurse can be a ladylike woman under all circumstances, and the good example of the one nurse will help some other nurse to hold to her highest ideals of conduct. A nurse who is interested in the tone and reputation of the school can call the attention of other nurses to undignified actions which should be corrected. She can refuse to belong to that class of people known as "the quiescent good."

"Eleven apostles, working men, and a twelfth added in a later season, took up the Master's work, and made the world over new" says a popular writer. "If they had belonged to 'the quiescent good' nothing would have happened." Continuing, this writer asks, "What can you and I do to make our world a better place than it is? Merely good intentions will not overcome bad practices nor improve conditions. Conditions grow worse, frequently, because good people do nothing." The "quiescent good" members of a school can often be roused to work for better moral standards, if one nurse musters courage to quietly protest against practices which are lowering the whole tone of the school.

The responsibility for maintaining a proper tone in the schools falls much more heavily on the members of the intermediate and senior classes of a school than on the juniors. Probationers and juniors are very apt to copy the bad as well as the good habits of their seniors. Every nurse who indulges in habits or practices which are undignified or vulgar, or in remarks which are flippant "slangy" or coarse, is helping to lower the moral tone of the school, and making it harder for younger nurses to live up to the best that they know.

Two probationers, who entered a church hospital school for training about the same time, were greatly shocked at the prevalence of profane language among the pupils of the school. If they had ever heard of the commandment "Thou shalt not take the name of the Lord thy God in vain" they were evidently failing to apply it in their daily conversation. Such expletives as "Good Lord," or "My God," and others of similar type, were disgracefully common. When the nurses were asked what the principal thought of the profanity, the probationers were told they had better not let her hear them using it. They decided that they would use their influence to stop this pernicious habit which they, later, found had begun with the entrance of one attractive, popular, but rather reckless nurse, now in her senior year. The course they decided on was to quietly ask every girl they heard using such language to please not take the name of the Lord in vain. The simple fact of calling attention to this evil was sufficient to check the habit in most of the nurses who indulged, and within a year the use of such language had died out in that school. This kind of influence quietly and tactfully exerted will accomplish what no principal could hope to accomplish by many lectures and reprimands.

Treatment of Probationers.—One of the tests of character which comes to every nurse, comes in the attitude or manner which she assumes toward probationers and juniors. It is natural that seniors should feel just a little above the juniors, and that the juniors should take on little airs of superiority because they happened to enter for training a few months before the probationers, but it is not necessary that these airs of superiority should develop into harshness. It is not necessary that probationers endure the snubbing that was so common years ago. It is essential for the highest good of the school that every nurse radiate that spirit of helpfulness and kindness which should permeate every institution for the care of the sick.

There are numerous little methods which a kind-hearted thoughtful nurse may use who has not forgotten the bewilderment and depression of the first few weeks of her probation period, that will do much to lessen that horrible feeling of loneliness and timidity which a probationer feels, in a strange place, where she is on trial, and under close observation. Even the experience of going to the first meal in a nurse's dining room, where the probationer is keenly conscious that she is being "sized up" and commented on by the assembled nurses is an ordeal to most probationers. This experience can easily be rendered a more pleasant memory if nurses will only take the trouble to be kind. To call for the probationer, conduct her to the dining room, and see that she is treated with the courtesy due to any stranger and that she finds her way back to her room again, is a small service but one which will surely be gratefully remembered. Most people intend to be kind, and are willing to be kind, provided they happen to think about it, but the trouble with nurses as with many other people is that they often fail to perceive in such circumstances as the one just described, an opportunity to show personal kindness to a stranger. If we have within us the spirit of the Great Teacher, and are keenly desirous of helping all with whom we come into contact, we will not neglect these small courtesies to the stranger who has entered the training school household. If we study His wonderful life we will find that many of His wonderful deeds of healing were done "as he passed by" on some other errand. The opportunity to do this deed of kindness came, and He did not neglect it.

Things to Avoid.—Pages might be written by nurses as to things to be avoided by intermediates and seniors in their treatment of probationer and junior nurses, and the writing of some of them should prove a wholesome exercise for every class. A few "don'ts" are suggested here as illustrations of what to avoid. Every nurse of a year's experience should be able to make her own list.

Don't forget how awkward and strange you felt during the first few days in a training school.

Don't think it is clever to "scare" the new probationers by telling them all the weird and gruesome stories of hospital life you can think of.

Don't regard the presence of a probationer in your ward as an unmitigated nuisance. Every trained nurse was once a probationer.

Don't impose on probationers by asking them to run errands for you and do unattractive duties which you yourself are responsible for.

Don't forget that the spirit of loyalty to an institution, its methods and rules is contagious, and that your attitude toward these things will help greatly toward maintaining the desired tone in the school. Try to add a dozen additional "don'ts" to this list.

Misunderstood Rules.—In every school there are rules the reason for which is not understood at the beginning of the training period. One rule which generally prevails is the rule which forbids pupil nurses from visiting doctors in their offices, or from consulting with physicians about personal ailments without first consulting the principal of the school about the indisposition. This rule is often resented as a curtailment of personal liberty. Give reasons why such a rule is a necessity for a well-ordered school.

A young principal of a small hospital school neglected to announce or enforce such a rule. A probationer arrived, and before the principal was aware of it she had consulted three different physicians who visited the ward she was in about a gynecological ailment which she had. This nurse regarded her presence in a hospital as an excellent opportunity to get all the medicine and medical advice she wanted gratis. When the principal discovered this tendency in the nurse, she talked seriously with her about it. The nurse persisted in the practice when she thought she would not be discovered, and of talking over her personal ailments with doctors whenever and wherever she chose. In other respects she proved an acceptable candidate. Was this proclivity in this probationer a sufficient reason for rejecting her?

A principal on assuming charge of a school found that one of the visiting doctors was in the habit of making visits after ten o'clock at night, and of spending an hour or more in "visiting" with the senior night nurse who was serving as night supervisor. After this nurse came off night duty, she paid frequent evening calls to this same physician in his office. When asked the reason for these visits, she stated that the doctor was treating her for headache and throat trouble. The nurse had completed all but about five months in a three-year term of training. What effect on the tone and reputation of the school will this nurse's conduct have? What should the principal of the school do in regard to this matter?

Hasty Judgments.—There is perhaps no more common failing among pupil nurses than their tendency to criticize the motives and decisions of the principal of a school, to proclaim that she has been harsh and unjust in dealing with certain pupils, when they have but a half knowledge of the real facts in the case. Tempests in schools are often worked up, serious issues are created out of mistaken sympathy for some pupil who is suspended or dismissed and deserved to be, but who protests her absolute innocence and purity of motive. The pupils often fail to take the larger view of the good of the school as a whole, and perhaps after keeping up a seething discussion of the principal's actions come in a group to the training-school office, asking that the dismissed pupil be reinstated.

It is well never to lose sight of the plain rule of justice that if a privilege could not wisely be allowed to forty or one hundred nurses, it should not be allowed to one pupil. Keeping this rule in view helps wonderfully to steady conditions in turbulent times.

A certain third-year nurse in a small hospital was placed in general charge on night duty. Two junior nurses were on duty on the second and third floors, the charge nurse being on the main floor. She developed a flirtation with the policeman in that district, and was in the habit of entertaining him for a longer or shorter time each night in the hospital, frequently serving refreshments. The junior nurses were cautioned to say nothing about it. However, the offense was discovered and the nurse was dismissed. Was the dismissal justifiable?

What would be the effect on the reputation of the school and the welfare of the patients if all pupil nurses were allowed to do as this nurse did?

Suggested Subject for Written Work.—What are some

of the reasons why a nurse's conversation with doctors and internes should be limited to professional affairs while on duty?

QUESTIONS FOR DISCUSSION OR REVIEW

1. What should a nurse do when a middle-aged respected member of the visiting staff is inclined to be just a little too familiar, not shockingly improper, but indiscreet?

2. What should a nurse do when a doctor tells in her presence a story which is intended to be a joke, but which is coarse, vulgar and decidedly "off color?"

3. How may a nurse keep to a sensible middle course and avoid being prudish on the one side, or on the other side drift into loose habits of conversation with professional people? How shall she avoid the criticism of being "gay" on the wrong subjects?

4. To what extent does a woman set the pace for a man in maintaining proper relations, or to what extent does she control the situation?

5. Explain what is meant by the phrase "tone of the school."

6. What responsibility has the individual nurse regarding the tone of the school?

7. Mention some things which intermediates and senior nurses should avoid in their treatment of probationers.

8. What bad effects in a school are liable to grow out of hasty judgment on the part of pupils in regard to the principal or head nurse?

9. Show how the rule requiring pupils to report their ailments to the principal before seeking medical advice is a safeguard to every nurse.

10. Outline briefly some points which nurses should be careful to observe in dealing with male patients.

CHAPTER XIV

Ethical Aspects of Hospital Accidents

When Florence Nightingale, after her return from the Crimean war, began to call attention to the need of reform in the care of the sick, she announced that one of the very first requirements in a hospital is that it should do the sick no harm.

It is still necessary to call attention to that fundamental requirement in the hospitals of today, and to emphasize it still further by saying that the first requirement in a nurse is that she also should do the sick no harm.

From the very nature of their work, hospitals are places where accidents are liable to occur. They are devoted to the care of individuals who are not normal and who, in many cases, are not accountable for injury which they may inflict on themselves. Nurses, in common with other hospital workers, have to do their work under these conditions. They have to accustom themselves to the constant thought that an important part of their work is to prevent accidents, to prevent patients injuring themselves or each other, and also to see to it that no patient receives bodily harm through their inadvertence or neglect.

The term "accident" in hospitals, as ordinarily used by the public, suggests the idea of an injury caused by the recklessness, carelessness, ignorance, or negligence of some individual. While accidents of many kinds occur in hospitals, there are four classes which stand out conspicuously because of their frequent occurrence:

1. Burns due to hot-water bottles or other articles used for the external application of heat.
2. Mistakes in the use of drugs.
3. Delirious patients jumping from hospital windows.
4. Accidents connected with hospital elevators.

Every accident has both a legal and an ethical aspect. The legal aspect relates especially to the existing laws dealing with such accidents, and the extent to which the person responsible for the accident is liable for damages should the injured patient go to the courts for redress. The ethical phase concerns itself chiefly with questions of neglect of duty, and the responsibilities which should voluntarily be assumed by an individual whose negligence or ignorance has resulted in injury to another.

Because a hospital exists as a result of the altruistic motives of its founders, and because it is engaged in benevolent work designed to promote the comfort and general welfare of the public, it is less liable to suits for damages than institutions or concerns promoted for commercial purposes. It is only in comparatively rare instances that injured patients are able to collect damages from hospitals, yet the publicity resulting from accidents which are followed by court proceedings damages the hospital itself in the minds of the public. It has reacted to the disadvantage of many institutions by creating prejudice or distrust as to its management in the minds of people who are contributing to its maintenance or who were planning to make bequests in favor of the institution.

Justice requires for every pupil nurse that early in her career her attention be called by those responsible for her instruction to the need of extreme caution, the necessity of always being on the watch to prevent mistakes and accidents, and to the places where accidents are most likely to occur. She should be warned, but it depends on the nurse herself whether she heeds the warning, whether she pays careful attention to what is said to her and governs herself accordingly.

Carelessness is a term having many shades of meaning. Webster defines "careless" as "heedless; inattentive; unconcerned; unmindful; without thought or purpose; incautious; inconsiderate; remiss; not taking ordinary or proper care." There are degrees of carelessness. Most accidents occur not because the nurse is wilfully careless, but *because she is not sufficiently careful.* She is willing to take a risk. It is this willingness to take risks, this neglect to use the precautions which have been taught, that results in many accidents for which nurses are responsible. Occasionally a serious accident occurs because a nurse did not understand the order, and this emphasizes the necessity of every nurse making sure, before doing a thing, that she understands what she is expected to do and how to do it. But it must be admitted that too many accidents occur not because nurses cannot understand orders, but because they do not carefully read the orders, or because while they were reading the order they were thinking of something else.

Burns occurring in newly operated patients while unconscious from anesthetics, by nurses failing to exercise due precaution in regard to hot-water bottles, have occurred probably more frequently than any other kind of hospital accident. The ethical aspects of this accident are far too little considered. The nurse is reprimanded or disciplined in some way, but that does not undo the fact that damage has been done, or that patients frequently suffer other injuries when such burns are inflicted.

A patient, a railway mail clerk earning $80 a month, entered a hospital for a minor operation. The doctor told him he would be able to leave the hospital in a week or less, and able to be at his work in ten days or two weeks. The patient paid a substitute to take his work and expected to pay his doctor. He paid $15 a week in the hospital. The wound healed promptly, but he received a severe burn while unconscious from ether, a burn which was very slow in healing. The nurse responsible for the burn decided to say nothing about it when she discovered it. Through lack of care the wound became infected, and the patient had to remain in the hospital over four weeks. Instead of his hospital expense being $20 to $30, it was $70. His doctor's bill was correspondingly increased. He was obliged to pay a substitute for more than five weeks instead of one or two weeks and, in addition, he had to pay the rent of his room in a rooming house during the whole period he was in the hospital. Thus it will be seen that the carelessness of the nurse was directly responsible for the young man's loss of over $100, besides the bodily injury inflicted. What reparation should the nurse make, or the hospital make, for this violation by the nurse of the fundamental ethical principle emphasized by Florence Nightingale that a hospital should do the sick no harm? Thus ethical problems growing out of hospital accidents might be enumerated indefinitely.

An illustration of accidents which result from pupils not understanding orders occurred in an English hospital. The details were as follows: A probationer of a few weeks' experience was told to cleanse the heads of two patients, and if necessary to rub in carbolic oil. The oil which was commonly used for such purposes was a mixture of nine parts of olive oil to one part of carbolic acid. The probationer, instead of using the mixture, rubbed pure carbolic acid into the hair of a child of thirteen years who was waiting an operation for adenoids. The child died shortly after, before a doctor could be secured. The jury blamed the probationer for not using proper care, the head nurse for laxity in supervision of the probationer's work, and the superintendent of the hospital for allowiug pure carbolic acid and strongly poisonous drugs to be kept in the same cupboard with common medicines.

Who was most to blame?

An illustration of an accident of a different kind recently reported from a Berlin hospital shows the tragic consequence to the nurse herself, because of a mistake in the use of drugs the dangerous nature of which she fully understood. This also shows how long familiarity with the use of drugs may cause one to grow less cautious in handling them.

A schoolboy of fourteen was about to undergo a minor operation. Cocaine was used to deaden the pain. The nurse, whose duty it was to administer the anesthetic, dipping the hypodermic syringe by misadventure into the wrong bottle, injected a cocaine solution of 20 per cent. instead of 2 per cent. The lad expired almost immediately, and the nurse took the tragic consequences of her error so much to heart that she immediately injected into herself the fatal mixture, and died so suddenly that it was at first thought that she had succumbed to a heart attack. She had been employed at the hospital for fifteen years, and was regarded as one of the most trustworthy assistants on the staff. It is said that the two cocaine solutions were kept in precisely similar bottles, which stood quite close to one another.

Who was to blame for this double tragedy? What precautionary measures might have prevented it?

Accidents with drugs have frequently happened during the progress of building or alterations when the general order of things was disturbed and there was more or less confusion in regard to where solutions or medicines were to be placed. In a hospital in one of the central states, during alterations in the building, a nurse gave two patients on the same morning a half glass of a solution of bichloride of mercury, instead of a solution of magnesium sulphate. Both patients died. The solution bottles were exactly the same size and stood side by side, the labels being turned to the wall. Under ordinary conditions the bottles were kept on separate shelves.

The psychological effect on a patient who has had a wrong dose of medicine administered, even when the medicine was simple and harmless, is often most disastrous. Patients frequently refuse to believe that serious damage has not been done, and court proceedings have frequently been begun to recover damages from a hospital because of supposed damage to the "lining of the stomach" or to other internal organs, due to the mistake of the nurse in administering a medicine intended for some other patient.

A dim light where medicines are kept or measured, a blurred or indistinct label, and a careless method of labeling are all contributing causes to mistakes in the handling of drugs.

Fatigue and Confusion.—Experience has shown that many accidents in the handling of drugs occur during the busiest hours when nurses are hurrying to get through and off duty at a given time. Experience has also taught that a nurse needs to be especially on guard at those hours.

Quite frequently one very troublesome patient, who is making incessant calls on the nurse while she is trying to attend to other patients, will so confuse her mind that she neither thinks nor sees clearly. Excessive fatigue has the same effect. Fatigue itself is one of the laws of growth, but excessive fatigue is unwholesome and dangerous. A tired mind affects working efficiency. It is not possible always to guard against excessive fatigue, but it is well to know that it exposes a worker to real danger. This condition of confusion and exhaustion at the end of a day often results because a nurse "dawdled" over duties at the beginning, because she left till the end of the day duties which might have been done with ease several hours earlier.

General Precautions.—In the handling of drugs there are several general precautions which experience has shown to be necessary to be shown to all nurses, which if generally observed would go far to prevent accidents.

1. Remember that there is an element of danger in every drug.

2. Read your orders carefully and be sure you fully understand the order and the method to be used before you carry it out.

3. Never give or use a drug of any kind that is not plainly labeled.

4. Never give a drug in the dark or in a dim light.

5. Always read the label twice before pouring out the drug. Read it again before giving it.

6. Keep your mind on the work in which you are engaged.

7. Measure the dose carefully. Never guess at quantities.

8. Never give a pill, capsule or tablet which has accidently escaped from its container.

9. Never jump at conclusions in regard to fractional doses. Mistakes in the arithmetic of drugs may be fatal.

10. Never give a dose of medicine that you have a

shadow of doubt about. Omit the dose if you are not sure. Always remember that it is better to be sure than sorry.

Infections.—In the operating room and all through the hospital the nurse is peculiarly responsible for the prevention of infection. Frequently, while apparently exercising all due precaution in the operating room, she may err through ignorance or carelessness, or from failing fully to grasp the extent of her responsibility.

A patient entered a hospital for an operation for double hernia. The operating room supervisor was away and a senior nurse was in charge of the operating room, handling dressings, etc. Gloves were not then as commonly used as now. The nurse in charge had neglected to use the healing hand lotions provided by the hospital, and the ordinary precautions for keeping her hands in good condition, and her hands had become exceedingly sore.

The hernia wounds suppurated, and for a time it looked as if the results of the operation would be completely undone by the infection of the wounds. Every avenue by which a clean wound could have become infected was investigated, and in the investigation it developed that the nurse's hands, because they were sore, had not been properly scrubbed or disinfected. She said nothing about them because she was afraid of being taken from the operating room where she was most eager to stay. The patient's stay in the hospital was more than twice as long as it would have been if the wounds had not become infected, and the expense was correspondingly increased.

This is a case where a nurse allows her own eagerness to be in the operating room to imperil the safety of the patient, and is a distinct violation of ethical principles and the Golden Rule. The subject of infection as it relates to nursing practice is one which affords ample scope for ethical as well as technical failures.

Injuries to delirious patients who escape from hospital windows are not always the result of carelessness on the part of the nurse. They are as frequently the result of the management of the hospital which neglects to provide safety screens for windows of rooms in which such patients are confined. The nurse's responsibility in the tragedy which results comes frequently because of her disobedience to orders. She is told that she is not to leave the patient alone, even for a minute, that he is liable to injure himself, and that she must call another nurse to watch whenever she is obliged to leave the room. She *intends* to do this, but perhaps the other nurse does not respond promptly to her call; she disobeys orders and takes a risk, and the death of the patient results.

Should a nurse be punished for her part in this tragedy? If so, how?

Patients with suicidal intent are frequently admitted to hospitals and the nurse in charge of such carries more than ordinary responsibilities. In order that nurses may realize their personal responsibility more fully in regard to such patients, some institutions issue a card with a form somewhat like this:

(Name of Institution).

You are asked to take notice that patient, John Doe, Room No. —, is suicidal.

He has threatened suicide frequently by poisoning.

He has attempted to drown himself.

He must be kept under observation constantly.

Signed, A. B., Superintendent.

I have read the above warning and understand my responsibility.

Signed by all nurses who will have him in charge.

Another safety system in dealing with such cases is to issue a small disc or tag, on which is written the patient's name. The nurse who has possession of this disc is held responsible for the patient's life. If the nurse has to leave the patient even for a moment she surrenders the disc to another nurse who is responsible in her absence. The carrying of such responsibility is a severe test of the makeup of the nurse, and of her ability to be trusted with other large responsibilities.

Suggested Subject for Written Work.—Mention four or more kinds of accidents that commonly happen in hospitals, with rules or suggestions for their prevention which nurses should observe.

FOR DISCUSSION OR REVIEW

1. Mention an important requirement in the care of the sick that was emphasized by Florence Nightingale.
2. Give reasons why accidents are very liable to happen in hospitals and why eternal vigilance is needed to prevent their occurrence.
3. Describe three kinds of accidents to patients that you have observed in a hospital, telling how each might have been prevented.
4. Differentiate between the legal and the ethical aspects of hospital accidents.
5. What course should a nurse pursue who discovers that she has given a wrong dose of medicine to a patient?
6. If she believed the medicine given was simple and harmless, what should she do about it? Should the patient

be told? If so, who should tell him if he didn't know of the mistake? How is a nurse to know that a medicine is harmless?

7. Show how accidents in the handling of drugs frequently occur.

8. What suggestions would you make in regard to methods of labeling or placing drugs that would lessen the liability of mistakes occurring?

9. Show how a nurse's mistake in arithmetic may cause the death of a patient.

10. Why is it a principle of safety to pour medicine from the side of the bottle opposite the label?

11. State the precautions which you observe in giving medicines.

12. Outline the ethical responsibility of the nurse in the operating room.

13. Of what value is a good conscience in a surgical nurse to the hospital? To the patient? To the nurse herself?

14. Is a nurse responsible for accidents occurring through her ignorance if she had been told of necessary precautions but had not heeded what was taught her?

CHAPTER XV

Developing a Symmetrical Life

The purpose of these studies from the beginning has been to help nurses to study the nature and laws of personal life, the moral or ethical life of each individual nurse, and its relation to nursing and nursing problems; to help nurses to see, in well-balanced relation, the things that are true and right in personal life; to help them to steer their course along safe moral lines, amid the difficulties and perplexities that beset them in a nursing career.

Fourfold Nature.—A fact which should never be forgotten is that, apart entirely from obtaining a nursing education and experience, every nurse while in training is developing a life. To direct and develop this life so that she emerges from the training school a symmetrical well-balanced woman with a wholesome outlook on the world in general, and with right ideas as to the part she is to play in the world, is an important part of the training process. It depends to a considerable extent on the nurse herself whether she accomplishes this or not. Every nurse has a fourfold nature to be cultivated and developed. She has a physical, mental, spiritual, and social side to her make-up, all needing due care and cultivation, and the possibilities of becoming warped and stunted in growth, of becoming one-sided and narrow, are present in every nurse's life.

In a previous chapter a quotation from an address by Dr. Richard Cabot is made, in which he calls attention to the danger of narrowness as one of the great dangers which beset the profession, and all who know anything of nurses and nursing today are likely to agree with him as to the seriousness of this peril.

Ethics and Conversation.—By far the most frequent complaints about the trained nurse, in general, after graduation are these:

1. She requires too much waiting on.
2. She does not keep sacred her patient's affairs.
3. She talks "shop" incessantly.

In too many cases her conversation is devoted largely to discussing her previous "cases" or things relating to the world of sickness. It rests with each nurse to decide whether the public whom she serves can justly make such complaints about her. If a nurse stopped to ask herself the question: "What effect is my conversation likely to have on the mind of my patient," is it not probable that many things she talks about would be omitted? If she asked herself the question: "Will this bit of gossip, or this incident I am going to relate, have a tendency to brighten the day for my patient, to relieve the depression of sickness, to take his mind away from the realm of sickness and give him new and helpful interests, or will it help him to see the seamy side of life, will it add to the depressing state of mind which he already has to combat," is it not possible that many things which nurses talk about in the presence of their patients would be barred from a nurse's list of topics?

The influence of mind over body is generally recognized. We all have seen its results, and have had some degree of experience that has taught us the simple lesson that the state of mind, the things one thinks about do exercise a powerful influence over the bodily functions.

An individual hears something that surprises or offends and the color of his skin changes; he blushes. The capillary vessels in the face and neck dilate and a hyperemia results. The physical change has been directly due to the thought that came to his mind.

We have seen people ready with a splendid appetite to partake of a meal, when a disturbing bit of news arrives, news of the illness or death of a relative perhaps, and at once the body loses its keen desire for food; the appetite has vanished.

A meal is eaten under the influence of distressing conditions, with anxiety filling the mind, and the glands that furnish the digestive fluid refuse to pour out their secretion; the food ferments, toxins are formed, and a train of miserable physical symptoms arise, if the anxiety and worry continue.

We see a child who is hurt run to its mother, crying with pain. The mother kisses the spot, says a few comforting words; the mental state of the child has changed and the pain has gone. Thus illustrations might be multiplied to show what we all know to be true, that mental conditions powerfully affect the bodily functions.

The influence of mind over mind is quite as real as the influence of mind over body. We may not fathom the deep secrets of psychology, but we do know that our own mental state is actively influenced by the people that we associate with. A friend with a happy optimistic temperament meets us, and he radiates the same feeling. He refuses to cherish gloomy forebodings, sees much that is good and beautiful in the world, maintains a quiet confidence in the Infinite One, and in some inexplicable way his attitude of mind is communicated to us. A fussy, nervous individual makes it impossible to get into a tranquil, restful state of mind while in his presence. Those who are well and active in the affairs of life are able to better resist such influences than are invalids who are shut in by the four walls of a sick-room, and nurses should constantly remember that a good nurse ministers helpfully to the whole individual.

If it were possible for nurses to separate the minds and souls of their patients from their bodies and nurse only the bodies, it would matter little what a nurse talked about in the presence of the sick, but since she is expected to minister to the whole patient, his mind as well as his body, it does matter a great deal whether the thoughts the nurse arouses in him are constructive or destructive in their influence over the bodily functions.

A Battle with the Blues.—A gentleman who was about to employ a special nurse for his wife while she was in the hospital, requested especially to be given a nurse who would not discuss operations, or hospital affairs, or patients that she had previously nursed. The principal assured him that the nurse he would have would not inflict any of her experiences with operations, or patients, or in hospitals, on his wife, who was suffering from the mental depression following a long illness. The nurse was warned, and did not dwell on these topics to any great extent, but she had had some unfortunate experiences with men; she firmly believed that men in general were bad, and she tried to make her patient believe the same thing. All men she said were unchaste and impure in their personal lives, only their wives refused to believe it in many cases. She was simply obsessed with the idea of the iniquities of all individuals of the masculine gender; there were none good, no, not one! and this fixed idea injected itself into her conversation at every opportunity. It is unlikely that the nurse herself was conscious that she was allowing herself to dwell on this phase of life to such an unwise extent, or that she knew that her influence over her patient's mind was morbid and unwholesome, but a nurse should think and should know whether the thoughts that she thinks and expresses, are likely to fill her patient's mind with the joy of living, to help her to look out on a sunnier world, to deepen her faith in God and man, to add to her happiness or whether they will have the opposite effect.

The possibilities of the power of thought are tremendous, and no nurse can afford to let this potent force in the sick-room run riot. It is entirely within a nurse's power to refuse to harbor unpleasant thoughts, or to dwell on the sad and painful experiences of life. She can deliberately determine that her business in life is to exercise a constructive influence on her patient's mind, rather than a depressing destructive influence. She certainly can refrain, if she wills to do it, from inflicting the story of her own unpleasant or harrowing experiences on a helpless patient who cannot escape from her presence.

The Value of New Interests.—The best way to combat the tendency to form habits of gossiping about matters relating to the world of sickness, is to keep up a wholesome interest in the world outside, and, from time to time, to acquire new interests in life. Time for reading is limited while in training, but fifteen minutes a day or less spent in scanning the chief events chronicled in the daily papers, will serve to keep a nurse posted as to the progress of the important developments in her own community and country. An hour a week with magazines which give a review of world progress, will wonderfully widen a nurse's outlook on life. Then there are numerous great movements for social and moral uplift in our own land, which touch the nursing field at many points, movements which are opening new doors of opportunity for nurses every year, movements which nurses in training should know something about, such as the child labor movement, the playground movement, the great public health movement, the various forms of social service which are being carried on in the interests of immigrants, etc.

One of the easiest and most natural ways that a nurse can use to keep out of the ruts of monotony in thought and conversation is to maintain her relationship with some church, attend its services as regularly as possible and try to keep in touch with what her own church is doing at home and on foreign fields. No study that a nurse can engage in will do more to broaden her horizon and quicken her sympathies than a study of the modern acts of the apostles who are at work in foreign fields or in difficult parts of the home land. The nurse who desires this kind of culture can (for fifty cents or less a year) have any one of a dozen magazines come to her monthly that will bring to her stories of heroism and achievement in other lands, that will lead her out into new lines of thought and endeavor, and that will wonderfully enrich her personal life. From such a magazine one catches glimpses of the manners and customs of people in non-Christian lands, of their social and sanitary condition, their educational methods, of the great need for trained women in those lands, of what women from the western lands are doing to lift the burdens from women in oriental lands, and free them from the bondage of pernicious ancient customs. Nurses are having a wonderful part in this great movement. They are teachers of sanitary science, of home economics; they are bringing to the oppressed and down-trodden women, who, in many lands are considered simply as chattel property or as slaves, the inspiration, instruction and nursing care they have so long needed, and are helping to create in those countries a higher idea of the value of woman, and of her place in national life. No nurse who wishes to be known as a well-informed or cultured woman can afford to be ignorant as to progress in this great movement for the uplift of women that is going on all over the world, a movement in which the nurses of the future are destined to play a still more important part.

It was said of a certain group of women that "they knew of no great events to talk about, so they talked of small things as if they were great." The same could truthfully be written about many groups of nurses, who, during training, indulge in gossiping, endlessly, about their patients, at meals, in bedrooms, on street cars, and in public places, simply because they refuse to make the effort to direct their conversation into other channels of thought.

Conversational Standards.—Is it worth while to try to keep out of ruts in one's thinking and conversation? Is it worth while for a nurse to try to improve her conversational standards? If so, how shall she begin to do it? A good rule to start with is the following: "Whatsoever things are true, whatsoever things are honest, whatsoever things are just, whatsoever things are pure, whatsoever things are lovely, whatsoever things are of good report; if there be any virtue, and if there be any praise, think on these things."

Suggested Subject for Written Work.—What should a nurse do who does not desire to become a gossip, but who finds this pernicious habit of gossiping about patients' affairs, the short-comings of head nurses, habits of physicians, etc., prevalent among the nurses that she associates with? Can such a habit be stamped out among nurses? If so, how?

FOR DISCUSSION OR REVIEW

1. What is meant by a nurse's fourfold nature?

2. Mention three common complaints which the public make about graduate nurses.

3. Is it true that nurses cannot be trusted to keep their patient's affairs sacred? Give reasons for your answer. Can you be trusted?

4. Mention several ways in which a nurse may helpfully influence the mind of her patient and help her to combat the depression of illness; also subjects which she should avoid.

5. Write a brief paper on the influence of mind over body.

6. Can a nurse fix conversational standards for herself and adhere to them? Explain your answer.

7. Of what value to nurses are varied interests in life?

8. Show how a variety of interests tends to strength of character and is a safeguard to a nurse.

9. Prepare a list of books you would consider suitable to be read to the adult sick. Mention some kinds of books which should be avoided.

10. Can you think of any reason why a nurse should hesitate to attempt to read dialect stories aloud to her patients?

11. What sort of books would you consider suitable to be read to a sick child and give some precautions in regard to the reading which you would think necessary?

12. If a nurse desires to become proficient in story-telling, how shall she go about it? Are there any general rules to be observed that will contribute to the success of the story-telling effort? If so, what are such rules?

CHAPTER XVI

The Discipline of Daily Living

It is probable that no nurse ever appreciates the value of hospital discipline till years of experience with life and people have come to her. She does not appreciate how much it means in the building of her character that she is required and expected to be faithful, true, honest, fair to others; that her tendencies to grumble or criticize or gossip were repressed; that she was obliged to stick to her tasks, whether agreeable or not, till they were finished; that she had to be punctual; that she had to repress the hasty word she was about to speak; that she was given responsibility and expected to measure up to it.

Reliability.—The work of the world depends upon reliable people, and this is especially true of hospital work, where life and death issues often hinge upon some apparently small thing. "A reputation for being reliable is the key to most of life's successes. Friends, work, honor, all gravitate to the reliable person. Being reliable is not easy, surface work. It takes day after day and year after year of patient acceptance of responsibility, of picking up the threads that the careless drop, of being ready in emergencies where others fail, of doing uninteresting faithful work that others tire of and slight—it takes all this to make the dependable man and woman known and valued."

Honesty in Bedside Records.—In a previous chapter reference was made to the subject of honesty or reliability in a nurse's records. A nurse's bedside records are an index to her real character, an everyday test of her honesty. It is of small comfort to know that the records look well, are free from blots and erasures, etc., if they lie. The principal of a certain school relates the following experience in her school, an experience which is probably not confined to any one school.

On making rounds, unexpectedly, shortly before midnight she found that all the patient's records in a large ward were completed up till 7 A.M., with a few exceptions. Various patients were recorded as having had "a good night." Six ounces of milk had been taken by several at 2:30 and 6:30 A.M. and several had voided twelve ounces of urine at a certain morning hour. Digitalis had been given to one at 3 A.M. and whiskey to another at 5 A.M. Temperature, pulse, and respiration were charted at 6 A.M.

On another occasion a certain nurse in the same school had recorded a douche given to each of three patients for three successive nights, all of which douches were reported to have "returned clear." One of the patients complained of not having had her douche for several nights, and on inquiry the other patients stated that theirs, too, had not been given.

Another nurse in the same school recorded special tablets which were ordered for a patient each four hours, as given at 8 and 12, and that the patient was asleep at 4 A.M. when the tablet was not given. The facts were that the supply of these tablets had been exhausted and the head nurse had failed to have the stock renewed, and none had been given. This nurse was suspended for two weeks, and warned that if further dishonesty were discovered, she would be dismissed. In an inspection of her room, articles belonging to several other nurses were found in her possession.

How far can a nurse who is dishonest in her records be

trusted? What is her word worth? Will a nurse who will lie in her records be likely to be guilty of stealing also?

Adaptability, that quality so essential to a nurse's success, is being cultivated all through training. Whether a nurse learns the lesson, or develops this most desirable quality, depends greatly on her own attitude of mind, and her own temperament. She has the opportunity to acquire this quality of adaptability, if she really desires it.

One of the first tests that nurses have to meet, one which contributes considerably to the development of the quality of adaptability to varying circumstances, comes to her when she becomes a part of community life. She learns that there are regular hours for doing things, and that whether she is inclined to attend to them at the time ordered or not, she must do it. She realizes for the first time the importance of trifles. She protests at first against the existence of so many rules—rules as to what she must bring with her; rules about rising and retiring, about the condition in which she leaves her room in the morning, about when she must go to meals, about hair and clothing, about the shoes she wears; rules about when to stand and how to stand, and when to sit; about what subjects are proper to be discussed with doctors when on duty, when to speak and when to be silent; about what articles she may and may not put in the laundry; about a thousand things which she has exercised free choice about before she entered.

She learns that her tastes in food are not likely to be consulted, that she need not expect favors to be shown her, and that no one is likely to ask for her opinion about a multitude of regulations to which she is expected to conform, but she does not dream that she is cultivating adaptability through these conditions and restrictions. She learns meanwhile to submit herself to the will of others, to accept sweetly the restrictions of institutional living, to consider the rights and comfort and welfare of others of the same household, as of equal importance with her own.

Daily Discipline.—There is also the discipline that comes from carrying out, day by day, a more or less monotonous routine, which must often seem like drudgery. She needs to remember that no education is ever secured without drudgery, and that all work at times seems to the doer of it as real drudgery. Contact with suffering brings to a nurse a different sort of discipline from that which most workers receive and every nurse needs to guard against allowing firmness to degenerate into hard heartedness; to be careful in developing endurance, and self-control, that she does not lose some of the finer qualities which no nurse can afford to lose.

Some one has said that "there is such a thing as the prose of this world's work, even good work, eating like rust into the life; there is such a thing as the little daily cares rasping and fretting the womanliness and the godlikeness away until there is scarcely a sweet word left on the lips, or a noble thought in the heart. Every nurse has to guard against this. It is true she has to stand in the shadows with those who are in trouble, but her face can always be turned toward the sun, so that the true light may not only enable her to see her duty, but may beautify and ennoble it."

When a nurse has passed her first year of training, she should have grasped the principles that underlie the discipline which she perhaps protested against in the beginning, and should be capable of applying the best principles to her own character and conduct and life

If she will try to keep always in mind Florence Nightingale's idea that "nursing is God's business" she will find many duties made lighter; and she will find, what every nurse should try to find, a real joy in service.

Sympathy, that indefinable quality which is so much needed, and so quickly felt by patients and their friends, is better shown in deeds than in words. It has been defined as a fellow-feeling with others in their varied conditions of joy or grief. Sympathy is not a weak yielding to the whims of patients when such yielding will do harm. It is frequently shown in "humoring" a patient when it is quite permissible, but often not fully convenient to do so. While, as a general rule, sympathy is shown much better in deeds than words, yet there are occasions when nothing more remains to be done for the patient. All that one can do has to be done with the sorrowing relatives and friends who are feeling the first shock of their loss.

What can or should a nurse do or say under such circumstances that will impress the friends that she has a real feeling of sympathy with them in their loss? What can she do that will give them a crumb of comfort or satisfaction at such a time? What can she do, or should she do to interpret to those friends and relatives, the real feelings of compassion and human kindness that animated the founders of the hospital?

Reverence.—A nurse reveals her true character to a considerable extent, by her reverence or lack of reverence for sacred things, or for the solemnities of life and death. It is unfortunate that familiarity with death should so frequently rob nurses of that awe which should be felt in the presence of death.

What responsibility has a senior nurse who assists a junior for the first time in caring for a dead body? If your mother or sister or a near relative were about to die in a hospital, mention three things you would rightly expect of the nurse in charge, before death occurred, and three qualities you would expect her to manifest in her care of the body after death.

Faithfulness.—All nurses cannot be quick or brilliant. All cannot take the highest grade in examination, but all can be faithful, and there is no quality which means more to a nurse in meeting the stern tests of life, than the simple quality of being faithful to the trust reposed in one. A nurse can receive no higher commendation than "Thou hast been faithful."

The grumbling nurse is found at some time in all schools. She may be capable, and of more than average intelligence, but she is unable to adapt herself sweetly to the rules and restrictions necessary to the life and routine of an institutional household. She frequently is found, often before her probation period is passed, freely criticizing the methods and rules of the institution to other nurses. In the blind confidence born of inexperience and ignorance, she imagines she could manage the hospital or training school or department far better than those who have had years of experience. Such nurses grumble about rules, about work, about food, about duty hours, about one thing one day and another the next, till they succeed in keeping all with whom they associate uncomfortable. There is only one thing to be done in regard to a nurse of this type, who persists in grumbling and criticizing and stirring up discord that poisons the atmosphere of the place, and that is to get rid of her. The habit of grumbling in some people is chronic, and usually it is to a greater or less degree contagious.

It is well for nurses to remember that few if any principals are fully satisfied with the results of their management; that they are fully conscious of many conditions which should be improved, and are patiently waiting for the right moment to make some needed adjustment. They are not half so blind as some pupils suspect, but they have to depend on very human machinery for the working out of plans for improvements, which are often delayed from causes difficult to control. Very often the grumbling nurse, apart from her undesirable disposition, is an inferior, unreliable worker, one whom the principal would be very glad to be relieved of. The grumbling nurse sees a variety of things which she wants changed to suit her tastes; the principal sees perhaps a very inferior nurse who may not commit any flagrant crimes or misdemeanors, but who will never be a credit to the school, and who is likely to prove a disturbing element wherever she goes.

The nurse with a real grievance belongs to a different class. That, even in this twentieth century, nurses sometimes suffer from unnecessary and preventable discomfort, cannot be denied. Quite often the principal may be so overwhelmed with pressure of other duties, that she has not had the existence of the grievance impressed on her. There is too, a possibility of knowing a thing without having its full importance brought to one's attention.

What to do with a Grievance.—Very rarely is anything gained by airing one's grievances in corridors and bedrooms, with those who are in no position to correct the conditions complained of. There are two or three things which may safely be advised in dealing with grievances in general. First, be sure it is a real grievance and not a fancied one. Second, write a statement of the grievance on paper, and let it cool for a few days, or longer. Be sure it is not exaggerated. If it still seems a real grievance that can be and should be remedied, go in a quiet, ladylike, dignified way to the person in authority, who is in a position to correct the conditions complained of, and ask if something may not be done to improve matters.

It is well always to remember that the narrow outlook which a pupil nurse necessarily has as a result of working in one corner of an institution, and being unable to see the problems of the hospital or school as a whole, invariably has a tendency to lead her to magnify small grievances into large ones, to become irritated at trifles, which in later years will appear ridiculous.

If, after having done this, the grievance continues, what course should a nurse pursue? The old adage, "Better endure the ills you have, than fly to those you know not of," is a good one to remember. The courageous acceptance of such disagreeable conditions as nurses could not remedy, has had a large part in the making of the best nurses the world knows today.

Truth and Falsehood.—There is probably no ethical question which seems to a serious minded nurse more puzzling than the matter of telling the truth. From the beginning of her career she is impressed with the idea that in the eyes of many members of the medical profession, it is an unpardonable sin to lie to a doctor about a patient, but perfectly pardonable, and frequently very desirable, to lie to a patient about his own condition. Thus this "double standard" as to truth in medical affairs confronts a nurse and adds to the confusion of her own ideas of duty, all along the way.

"The great bulk of medical work, public and private, is still done by men, high-minded men, who believe that it is impossible to deal frankly and openly with patients,"*

* Social Service and the Art of Healing.

says Dr. Richard Cabot, in discussing the questions, "How far should we speak the truth in dealing with our patients, our colleagues, or anyone else? Are lies ever in place? If so, under what conditions?"

The substance of the teaching given in medical schools on the question of truth-telling in medical matters is summarized by Dr. Cabot as follows: "'When you are thinking of telling a lie,' said the teacher, 'ask yourself whether it is simply and solely for the patient's benefit that you are going to tell it. If you are sure that you are acting for his good and not for your own profit, you can go ahead with a clear conscience.' The lies which the medical profession agree in condemning are those told for personal and private gain."

Veracity is defined by the same writer as "doing one's best to convey to another person the impression that one has about the matter in hand." One may do one's best and yet fail, but that is not lying. A true impression, not certain words literally true, is what we must try to convey. By lying is meant an intentional deception, however brought about.

The Technic of Telling the Truth.—In answering the question as to whether the truth should be told when it may kill the patient, the writer quoted suggests that it is in very extraordinary and rare cases that a life could be saved by a lie, and that the nervous systems of patients and friends on whom the experiment has been tried of telling the truth about their condition when a lie would have been easier, have shown an amazing immunity from depressing effects. "It seems as if, when the pinch comes and the individual has to face stern realities, some species of antitoxin is spontaneously and rapidly developed whereby the individual is rendered immune to the effects of the expected shock."

The way in which a thing is told has so much to do with the way in which it is received, that all nurses need to study carefully the best way of putting disagreeable facts before a patient or his friends when asked for them, or when it is desirable for the facts to be known. See page 54. Is there such a thing as "a lie of necessity?" If so, give an illustration of such necessity.

Mental Therapeutics.—The wise use of "persuasion" and "suggestion" as therapeutic measures is advocated today by the best and most successful physicians. To many, the giving of placebos is simply a form of suggestion which they feel is perfectly justifiable. Instead of trying to persuade a patient or of using time and effort to impress a patient's mind with the idea that he will sleep tonight, thus creating in his mind the right mental conditions for sleep, they give a bread pill or a sugar of milk tablet and say, "This medicine will put you to sleep."

Placebos with or without lies, Dr. Cabot believes,* are unnecessary, unless in the very exceptional cases in which one is dealing with a foreigner or an individual who cannot understand the explanations given. He claims that the giving of placebos is fostering the patent medicine habit, and helping to educate the patient, and the public, to a harmful dependence on drugs, to a wrong idea of the way in which disease is produced and avoided, is helping to perpetuate false ideas about how health is to be secured and maintained. Do you agree with this opinion? If not, why not?

In the use of placebos, does the value of the suggestion depend on the patient not finding out that he has been deceived? Is it a good thing to have a patient's confidence rest on such a flimsy foundation as "not being found out?"

* Social Service and the Art of Healing.

In what way might the use of placebos help a patient to an unwholesome dependence on drugs, and induce a habit of drugging for every ailment?

What is meant by the use of "persuasion" and "suggestion" as therapeutic measures?

To what extent and in what ways may a nurse use these methods in her everyday practice?

Suggested Subject for Written Work.—Is it possible for every nurse to be a living demonstration to those who know her, that she is capable of doing the work of a true nurse in the world without losing any of the sweet and beautiful qualities we covet for all women. If you believe it is, show how it can be done.

FOR DISCUSSION OR REVIEW

1. What is reliability? How is it shown?
2. Of what value to a nurse is a reputation for reliability?
3. What value should be attached to dishonest bedside records?
4. What responsibility has a nurse who discovers that one of her associates is practising dishonesty in her records?
5. Is it dishonest to record a duty as done before it is done, when a nurse simply thinks she will do it?
6. Show how adaptability is cultivated in the everyday routine of a hospital.
7. Mention several ways by which a nurse may show her sympathy with a patient or his friends, and several methods of showing sympathy which she should avoid.
8. Explain in detail what is meant by reverent care for the dead.
9. When a nurse finds one of her associates inclined to grumble constantly, what should she do?

10. What is the best course for nurses to pursue who believe that they have a real grievance?

11. In a certain hospital there is a rule posted in the nurse's dining room requiring all complaints about food or the way it is served to be repressed while in the dining room, and submitted in writing to the superintendent. Would such a rule tend to greater comfort or discomfort during meal hours? Would it tend to lessen or increase grumbling about food? Why?

12. Prepare a list of suggestions by which the variety in institutional food might be increased without increasing the cost.

13. If you had to cater for fifty or a hundred nurses, what rules would you adopt in order to satisfy them all?

14. What is the best way to deal with a nurse who is a chronic grumbler and never satisfied?

15. Mention some examples of the successful use of "suggestion" used as a therapeutic measure by nurses.

CHAPTER XVII

Manner and Temperament

It is a common mistake in nurses to feel that in the first few months or a year they have acquired a good deal more knowledge than they really have, and to fail to realize how much there is yet for them to learn before they should be sent forth as trained women. They have not learned to distinguish between knowledge and wisdom.

Good judgment comes only as the result of experience and of a wider knowledge than any nurse can hope to acquire in a short time. Many nurses fail to remember that the self-control, the power of wise decision, the resourcefulness, the quickening of the powers of observation and perception, the complete reliability which makes a good nurse a tower of strength to an institution or household have to be patiently acquired; they cannot be learned from books, cannot be put on with the uniform, they cannot be purchased.

Many nurses bring with them certain mannerisms—ways of speaking or acting—which are more or less crude. They have sharp edges to their make-up, which training should help them to eradicate. Many "diamonds in the rough" are admitted for training in the hope that, through training, the fine qualities that are believed to be in them may be developed and the rough edges smoothed away. This process takes time and patience, not only on the part of the nurse herself, but probably a greater degree of patience on the part of those responsible for her training, who must meanwhile put up with the results of her crudeness, her lack of judgment, her foolish weaknesses, or her unfaithfulness. There are perhaps few failings in nurses that are more exasperating than the quality of self-complacency which so often develops after the first year's training has been finished.

Self-training.—It is hard for a nurse to comprehend that the acquisition of technical knowledge and the passing of examinations are but one phase of training, and that the change which she needs to have wrought in her is often much farther from being accomplished than she is able to realize. Nurses frequently come asking for a course of training when they do not desire training. They rebel against it. They would be satisfied with a certain very moderate amount of *instruction*. They act as if they expected to have technical knowledge poured into them as though they were empty vessels, with no inherent qualities that would prevent their retaining all that was taught. That they bring with them bad habits that must, if possible, be trained out of them, that they have weak points that need to be strengthened, and latent good qualities developed, all of which takes time, is a thought rarely grasped by a pupil on entrance.

Types of Nurses.—In every school there will be found nurses who seem to have no higher motive than simply to secure a diploma, and who wish to do as little as possible and study as little as they can possibly manage to get through with; who seem to be in no way desirous of correcting glaring defects in character, even when attention is called to them. Others are quick but superficial, content to slight their duties whenever it seems convenient, and have no aspiration toward thoroughness.

Another type is slow in grasping new ideas and methods, but make up for this in their faithfulness to details and their general loyalty to the welfare of patients and the institution. They quickly develop the quality of being "dependable" and impart a feeling of security and confidence wherever they are at work. Still another group of nurses demonstrate quickly their power of constructive thinking and planning. They manifest that quality known as "initiative." They see things to be done and do not have to be told every slight detail. They see things out of place and put them where they belong, without waiting to be told. They show a proper regard for hospital property and try to keep it in good condition. They are not given to wasting time in gossip, and get along well with their associates.

Describe some other types of nurses whom you know—nurses who will not fit into any of the classes mentioned.

Good Manners.—Of what value is a refined manner to a nurse? How will courtesy and good manners affect her success in life? How much responsibility have the training-school authorities to correct defects in table etiquette in nurses? In what ways can nurses help each other to acquire good habits and correct bad habits in the dining room and elsewhere?

Mention some common lapses in table etiquette which you have observed among nurses.

Is the habit of using slang likely to be a hindrance to a nurse? Mention common examples of slang or expletives which you have noticed nurses indulging in that you think might be a hindrance to a nurse in her professional life?

Two nurses who were friends before they entered for training persisted, in spite of orders to the contrary, in calling each other by their Christian names, and occasionally by such terms as "Dearie" and "Honey," while on duty. What are the chief reasons for objecting to this practice?

The stony manner so frequently used by fiction writers in portraying nurse characters is unfortunately not entirely an imaginary quality. It exists in far too many nurses, and the term "*stony lady*" used by a little girl patient in speaking of her nurse is far too apt a characterization of some nurses.

A writer in an English journal,* in commenting on this subject, says some plain things which are worthy of reflection by every nurse:

"The 'hospital manner' has become a by-word, and the profession which should be a model of gentle kindliness is often held up to just reproach on account of the abrupt discourtesy of its speech, the stiff aloofness of its manner, its want of sympathy and politeness as displayed to strangers or to subordinates.

"Constant daily association with strangers tends to make some natures silent, unresponsive, unsympathetic. Because they are strangers such people do not find it worth while to be pleasant, courteous, or genial. They go about their business self-contained and indifferent to others. When spoken to they are monosyllabic, abrupt, curt to the verge of rudeness. They ask but little of others and never go out of their way to do an unasked kindness to anyone. They may be of sterling worth under this hard crust, but their better qualities seldom find their way to the surface because of what the kind-hearted describe as their 'unfortunate manner.' These people sometimes become embittered because their good qualities and real ability remain unrecognized, while others, less reliable and not half as clever, secure some coveted post or easily win promotion or praise. They will not allow that the same good things might have fallen to their own share also had they only possessed

* Nursing Mirror.

equally gracious and pleasant manners. They pride themselves upon that very abruptness which hinders their advancement. They hug their curtness and call it sincerity; their rudeness and christen it truth.

"Surely, if any members of the community ought to cultivate good manners, nurses should do so. To them, rather more than to most, they mean success. At the very commencement of her career a well-mannered girl stands on a different footing from her more uncouth companion. Her fellow-nurses like her, the patients take to her, the head nurse of the ward sees in her a promising pupil, the principal is favorably impressed. As she goes on she finds difficulties smoothed by her invariable courtesy; she can bend patients, juniors, servants to her wishes; even members of committees yield to her charm of manner.

"*Good manners* ensure the immediate success of the head nurse, the superintendent, the private nurse, in all those countless intricacies of daily life which call for tact and courtesy. If they are indeed the 'fruit of a loyal nature and of noble mind,' then, when combined with ability and professional skill, it is safe to prophesy that the nurse possessing them will go far.

"True, it is difficult in the daily 'hussel and bussel'—as a little maid once spelled it—of hospital life to remember and practise always the grace of courtesy. The time goes so fast, interruptions are so numerous, and there are so many duties to claim our attention that almost before we know it the staccato note has crept into our voice, and we are nothing if not abrupt. People are deaf, people are stupid, and we are compelled to suffer fools, though not gladly. Thronging duties hem us in on every side until sometimes the common courtesies of life are allowed to slip from us unheeded. Yet some of the busiest of people have been noted for their good manners, while those possessed of ample leisure are not always the most courteous.

"The best manners have their origin in a kind, unselfish nature, a sympathetic mind, a feeling heart. They are the outcome of a spirit of reverence toward God and man, the expression of true benevolence, and, as Lord Rosebery has put it, 'a sign of charity toward your fellow-man, a part of your duty to your neighbor; they are also a sign of self-respect.'

"Good manners are not incompatible with sincerity. Nearly always there is something pleasant to say if we will only say it, just as true as, and infinitely more acceptable than, the abrupt word and unsmiling look. Courtesy establishes friendly relations at once and goes far to oil the wheels of daily life."

Temperament and Institutional Work.—The author receives numerous inquiries regarding nurses for institutional positions and always the matter of temperament is mentioned as one of special importance. If you were seeking for a principal or supervisor for a hospital school in which you were interested, what temperamental qualities would you desire to find? What other qualities?

The following description of a head nurse was written by a Turkish patient after an experience in a hospital in New York City. Analyze his description and compare it with your own ideal for a head nurse. What points did the Turkish patient overlook that should be embodied in the ideal you have in mind of what a head nurse should be temperamentally?

"I wish to speak especially for the head nurse. She seems so simple, so even, so obliging, so sympathetic and so kind a woman as I have ever seen. She creates a smile even if she had none. She makes a sympathy with every little complaint to her. She answers short and simple. She walks around scattering grace and peace everywhere. She gives one smile to a sufferer and to another a sympathetic nod. She is very kind to her nurses. She speaks obligingly (kindly, he means), but yet commands. She asks yieldingly, yet demands. She inquires beseechingly, yet compels. She is medium aged, modest looking, bright, fair complexioned, has a forehead which could show her intellect, a modest nose that may betray her great patience, a pair of eye-glasses behind which two glittering eyes which could tell that their owner had shaken hands sometimes with the messengers of every kind of misery and disappointment. Anyhow I must not go further for an American lady which is your national sister and my human friend. The other nurses I do not care for; they seem very greenhorns yet."

Special nurses for private patients in hospitals can be either a real help or a real detriment to a training school. Analyze the most nearly perfect "special duty" nurse whom you know, and try to decide what qualities she seems to possess that other nurses lack. What are the reasons why doctors and patients seem to prefer her, and why the hospital calls her in preference to some others?

Temperament and Private Duty.—If manner and temperament are important in filling a hospital position, they are even more so in private homes. Two types of nurses will illustrate this point. The nurse whose management of her cases is so plainly in evidence that everyone in the home is made uncomfortable is a type not infrequently met with. Such a nurse is described thus by a nurse writer:* "Miss H. is mentally alert and neatness personified. She was the valedictorian of her

* Helen Wilson in The Trained Nurse and Hospital Review.

class, but alas for her patients! She rules them as rigidly as if they were prisoners. She has what is called 'a commanding presence.' Everyone gets out of the way when she arrives. The poor miserable patient feels the shock of her arrival most of all. While she takes the temperature, pulse and respiration on the minute, she wears an air of stern seriousness.

"She takes a quick survey of her surroundings and plans her attack. The position of the bed is changed, and before she has been in the house half an hour, the hall is filled with articles considered superfluous and unhygienic. Her commanding presence is quickly felt in the kitchen, where the cook is given *freely* a course in domestic science. The doctor's orders are carried out to the letter; not one medicine or treatment is omitted." No one can call her lazy, but somehow every one heaves a sigh of relief when the door closes behind her. Can you tell why? Why is such a nurse not kept busy? Wherein was her failure? How far is it wise to try to discipline a patient when in a private home?

Another case in which manner causes the nurse's failure occurs somewhat as follows:

Dr. Blank calls a registry and asks for a nurse whom he knows for a mild case of nervous exhaustion. The nurse he asks for is busy, but the registrar sends another nurse, the one whose name is at the top of the registry list. The doctor expects the case to last at least two months, possibly longer. He wishes the patient to have complete rest in bed and to gain in weight. The remainder of the story is thus told by the writer quoted.

"The nurse arrives. She is the picture of health, tall, a perfect physique, and very pretty. She is dressed in the height of fashion, of a certain type. Her hat, the largest money could buy, is trimmed—it surely must have resembled David Harum's wife's bonnet, so nearly did it come to having 'glass beads and garden truck' upon it. It did have two very weather-beaten peaches and a bunch of grapes on one side and a willow plume on the other. Her flimsy black dress would have passed for an evening gown, so 'dutched' was the neck. She wore a gaudy necklace and numerous rings.

"When greeted by her patient's husband she exclaimed: 'Well, say, I would have came out by the ten o'clock, but I just missed it. Say, ain't this a peach of a place though?'

"When she appeared later in her pretty pink uniform and kerchief she was indeed a picture as she stood in her patient's door."

She greeted the patient with a volume of the latest slang, which at once settled her grade as a nurse in the patient's mind. In just two days she departed and another nurse was called. Technically there was no complaint about her work—she was willing to do anything she saw needed to be done for the patient's comfort.

Which of the two nurses just described would you wish to have hovering over you if you were really ill? To what extent was each nurse to blame for her manner? Would it be possible for either to change her manner? How would you convince either nurse that her manner was a hindrance to her? Can you see why such nurses are likely to swell the discontented class that is always complaining that there are too many nurses?

Executive Ability.—There is no one quality or combination of qualities so much in demand in nurses as that known as executive ability. Institutions are always seeking for nurses with executive ability and the "right temperament" to take charge of training schools and departments.

What is this thing which is so much in demand in nurses and how can it be cultivated? Is it a natural gift or must it be acquired? These are questions of real importance to nurses who desire institutional positions or other positions of responsibility in the nursing field.

Is the following a satisfactory definition of executive ability: the power to think and plan and do, with a fair measure of success, without the supporting help and direction of others?

How far, and in what ways, may a nurse acquire this power or ability while in training? How can she demonstrate that she has this ability?

The Carrying of Responsibility.—In the opening chapter of this book it was stated that the most important thing for a probationer to demonstrate in the trial period was her ability and willingness to measure up to such responsibilities as came to her. All through her life she will be judged and valued largely according to her ability wisely to assume responsibility and easily and effectively to carry it. This ability comes largely through experience, though many never acquire it to any great degree. The tendency in the age in which we live is to centralize responsibility, and to make it the chief characteristic of leadership. The importance of a place and the remuneration attached to it depend very greatly upon the amount of responsibility to be borne.

The failure of many nurses who have had excellent training and splendid opportunities can be traced either to the question of disposition or temperament, or to their inability to think systematically and clearly, to act independently, and to carry responsibility effectively.

Lack of courage to stand alone, to meet opposition or difficulties without being crushed, is another common cause of failure in otherwise well-equipped women.

They always seem to need someone to make up their mind for them on important questions, or to go ahead of them and prepare the way. They are afraid to have real convictions on any subject for fear of being disapproved of or misjudged, or of meeting opposition. Such nurses may fill a niche in the world; without doubt there is a place for them, but it is not a large or important place. Can you think of any other quality which is a substitute for courage? How is courage acquired?

Looking Ahead.—During a nurse's second year she should be able to take stock of her own character, temperament, and ability to fill some certain position in the nursing field. From your present knowledge of nursing conditions, which line of nursing service most appeals to you? Give reasons for your answer.

Suggested Subject for Written Work.—Prepare a description of the qualities you think a nurse who desires to have charge of a surgical department should possess. Mention the three qualities which to you seem most important.

FOR DISCUSSION OR REVIEW

1. Which of the four types of nurses mentioned in the early part of this chapter would you consider best adapted for institutional work? Give reasons for your answer.

2. Write a short paper telling how a nurse reveals in a hospital whether she has the grace of good manners, and of what value good manners will be to her in institutional work, in private work, in visiting nursing.

3. Show how good manners may be a help to a nurse whose work is chiefly with dispensary patients in the dispensary and in their homes.

4. How may a nurse guard against "the hospital manner" described in this chapter?

5. What temperamental and other qualities would you expect a successful visiting nurse to possess?

6. Make a list of the faults you have observed in special nurses which you think all nurses should avoid.

7. Explain the term "executive ability." How may it be acquired? How is it demonstrated?

8. Mention one important point by which a nurse's value in dollars and cents is rated.

9. Mention any quality which seems to you a substitute for courage.

10. What is the difference between having convictions and having opinions?

11. What is meant by the phrase "the courage of one's convictions?"

12. Why is it that some nurses have convictions and others do not? How much does one's early training have to do with convictions?

CHAPTER XVIII

Health, Recreation and Friendship

A nurse's health is her most important asset. However skillful she may be in her profession, she cannot hope to attain her highest success in any line of nursing activities if she is in a debilitated uncertain condition of health, liable to be incapacitated for the performance of her work every little while. Granted that she entered training with a sound physique and average normal resistive power, her health during training is, to a very considerable degree, in her own keeping. Many nurses forget that the subject of personal hygiene is not a theory simply to be studied in order to pass an examination. It is a practical thing to be applied in a hundred ways every day in the year.

Nearly every nurse, in common with other individuals, has some point in her constitution which is weaker than other points and liable to be easily affected; when she knows where her weakness is, it behooves her to govern herself accordingly. It seems to be self-evident that those who aspire to nurse the sick should themselves be healthy, and the desire to keep at one's maximum physically should be strong enough in every nurse to keep her on her guard constantly against the things which would undermine her health.

Infections.—It has been abundantly proven that most infections which occur in hospitals are the result of contact, this in opposition to the older theory that infections were chiefly air-borne. In many cases infections are the direct result of the neglect of necessary and well-understood precautions which nurses have been taught they should be careful to observe.

Mention several instances of such neglect which you have observed in nurses.

Diet.—It is along dietary lines that nurses err more frequently than anywhere else in matters of health. Too free indulgence in tea or coffee, or indulgence at wrong hours, nibbling at candy, cake, nuts, etc., in off-duty hours, night suppers in rooms are common causes of ill health among nurses in training, causes which they should have learned to guard against long before they entered for training. Any nurse who has lived twenty or more years with herself should know what she can eat with safety, and what she ought to avoid eating.

A nurse who was ill in bed with some gastric disturbance had a mild fever, and was ordered to be kept on a milk diet till the fever subsided. A friend, hearing of her illness, sent her a two-pound box of candy which she surreptitiously ate in less than two days, while she was supposed to be making an effort to get well.

Another nurse had been out for a walk and was caught in a heavy shower. She returned just in time to go on duty at night and donned her uniform without changing her wet shoes, stockings and skirts, working all night in these wet garments. She was subject to frequent attacks of sore throat, and next day was so ill that she was unable to be out of bed. A severe attack of tonsillitis followed, and later a heart complication developed. As a result of this illness she was obliged to be off duty three months.

These are common illustrations of violations of the simple rules of health which nurses fully understand.

Overstrain in nurses, with the resultant loss of equilibrium and disturbance of nerve balance, is usually due to a combination of causes. Loss of sleep which is long continued, insufficient exercise in the open air, digestive difficulties—these, combined with worry, are found to a greater or less degree in most cases. All nurses suffer from overstrain in the early weeks of their training, due to the mental and physical effort required in getting accustomed to new surroundings and duties, in trying to remember the multiplicity of new things that need to be grasped in the very beginning; due also to the needless expenditure of strength and energy, the lost motions and wasted steps in doing tasks that are unfamiliar. This period of overstrain passes away in a short time, and the nurse develops a higher degree of resistive power and endurance, in much the same way that an athlete develops muscular strength and skill.

Worry plays a much greater part in sapping the vitality than, probably, any other one cause. It is a veritable demon that robs life and work of its joys, poisons the nervous organism at its very centers, and affects the smooth harmonious working of the machinery of the body in a variety of ways. If diligent efforts are not made to combat it, worry soon becomes a habit of mind that lessens efficiency and reacts adversely on the nurse in more ways than can readily be mentioned.

Is worry a habit which a nurse can correct? If so, how is she to successfully combat this habit? A well-known American psychologist, Professor James, says: "The sovereign cure for worry is religious faith. The turbulent billows of the fretful surface leave the deep parts of the ocean undisturbed, and to him who has a hold of vaster and more permanent realities, the hourly vicissitudes of his personal destiny seem relatively insignificant things."

If one would avoid worry it is important to avoid doing things which are liable to lead to keen regrets or over-anxiety, and a nurse cannot too early learn this important lesson. This rule can be applied in a nurse's life in a thousand ways. When it comes to matters as to the wisdom of which there is room for doubt, it behooves a nurse to walk cautiously, if she is not to invite worry. Another wise rule is never to make an important decision when one is physically or mentally weary or depressed, or not in good condition physically. Many causes of worry are preventable if one uses reasonably good judgment.

*How to be an Optimist.**—Dr. J. H. Kellogg gives the following rules for those who would cure themselves of habits of worry:

"To cure worry you must cultivate hope; to cure pessimism you must deliberately cultivate optimism. You must force your mind into optimistic channels of thought. This can best be accomplished by reading optimistic authors and talking with optimistic people. A very excellent plan is to set yourself the task of curing some pessimistic person by deluging him with optimistic ideas and expressions. If the physical causes which were originally responsible for the morbid condition have been corrected, this habit of making mental sunshine for others will in the end produce an optimistic habit of thinking, and will become permanent, thus eradicating pessimistic thought habits by substitution.

"It is a well-known fact that the best actors often actually experience the emotions which they depict in their acting—when counterfeiting laughter, for instance, they often actually experience the thrill of good cheer which normally accompanies the act of laughing. There is, indeed, the most substantial ground for believing that one may not only form but reform his habits by deliber-

* Good Health Magazine.

ately producing through the will such mental and physical activities as are normally associated with mental and physical acts, the opposite of those of which it is desirable to rid oneself.

"If one feels reticent, disagreeable, and sullen, he may dissipate the evil spell by assuming an air of cheerful amiability and sociability quite different from the inward feeling, with the result that the mask of geniality will soon permeate the mind and character, and develop kindred habits of thought and action, and thus effect a cure.

"Remember, too, that fatigue has an important effect on the channels along which our impulses travel, with the natural result of weakening the resistance of the will against the undesirable contacts that result in wrong and unwise acts. A prolonged condition of fatigue is thus a source of great danger.

"A countless number of physical, mental, and moral disasters result from this weakening of the will resistance and the opening of the doors of impulse. To the tired brain, facts appear distorted. Values are displaced, sanctions are ignored, resolutions are forgotten, good intentions fly to the winds, impulse is in the ascendency, the senses predominate." A good holiday is often the best antidote for worry.

A few sensible health laws which a group of club women worked out for themselves, and which apply equally well to nurses are these: "To eat well, neither too much nor too little and of proper food; not to worry; to govern one's nerves, and maintain a steady faith in God; to play often; to laugh; to think much of others and little of one's self; to spend a part of every day in the open air; to be hopeful; to love both God and man; to look on the bright side of life; to have always some congenial work to do, some responsibility to carry, and whatever happens, to be good-natured."

Recreation.—Inseparably interwoven with the matter of health is the subject of recreation. The most splendid energy will flag, enthusiasm for one's work will wane, and the best balanced person will become irritable, unless there enters into one's life reasonable recreation. The human system demands change as well as rest, if it is to remain in good condition.

The choice of recreation, so that it really recreates, and gives new strength and enthusiasm, requires much judgment. Nurses in training, and after training, often show a woeful lack of good sense in regard to how they spend their off-duty periods and holidays. Many of them do not seem to know where recreation ends, and dissipation begins.

True recreation is best secured by a combination of three things; *change of air,* getting completely away from the hospital and training school, or the sick room, or one's work; *change of thought,* the banishing for the time everything connected with the care of the sick or nursing affairs; and *change of exercise and habits.* It is just as much a nurse's duty to learn to rest properly and wisely as it is to learn right methods of work. A proper amount of sleep and rest are a necessary part of recreation. In her efforts to secure what she thinks is recreation, a nurse too often becomes unnecessarily and unwisely fatigued, and returns to her work and studies worn out rather than refreshed. Long walks are taken; tiresome shopping expeditions are planned; errands are undertaken for other people; exhausting excursions are taken; late hours are indulged in; or perhaps, week after week, the nurse frequents moving picture shows in her afternoon off duty, instead of securing the variety in pleasure that she really needs. Every nurse with ordinary observing powers should be able to make out a list of things to be avoided in matters of recreation.

The annual vacation presents a different sort of problem from the short off-duty periods, and one which requires wise management by the nurse herself if she is to get the rest and benefit from it that every nurse needs.

A mistaken idea of duty and values often prompts a nurse to ask to be allowed to use her vacation in nursing friends or relatives, or in making up time lost by illness. Both of these plans have been found to be against the best interests of the nurse, and of the hospital. In many schools, rigid rules exist which require a nurse to spend her holidays in freedom from nursing of any kind, in real recreation, so that she can bring to the work of the year to follow a rested body, a clear mind, strengthened nerves, and fresh courage and enthusiasm.

Equally unwise has it been found in actual practice to allow nurses to take two years' vacation in one year. Shorter and more frequent periods of rest yield better results as a rule than longer vacations at longer intervals, but it is often difficult to make a nurse believe that what she wants in regard to her vacation is not always best. Quite often it will be found that the nurse whose health breaks down before her training is finished, or who finishes it in an utterly exhausted condition of body, has been most unwise in regard to the management of her sleeping hours, her off-duty periods and her annual vacations, or has been worrying over matters in no way connected with her work, while she poses as a martyr whose debilitated health is entirely due to her devotion to duty and to overwork.

Friendship.—The nurse who desires to maintain a true balance in her life, to avoid the danger of mechanical service, of narrowness, and numerous other dangers that are common to institutional life, will find that the friendships she forms during training will have much to do with the progress that she makes in various directions. Friends have much to do with the making or marring of both a nurse's happiness and reputation. They both reflect her character and profoundly affect it. The ancient proverb still is true that "a man is known by the company he keeps." A nurse's choice of friends will affect materially the confidence that other people impose in her and their general estimate of her as a woman.

Violent Friendships.—A mistake which many nurses make is in the formation of violent friendships on very short acquaintance, and with people of whose character they have but a superficial knowledge. Another mistake is that of allowing the feeling to develop that one's friend is an absolute necessity to one's happiness. It is only by sad experience that many nurses learn that friendship has its perils, very real perils, that sudden and violent friendships usually result disastrously, and that it is a mistake to attach one's self to one person so exclusively that one neglects to make other friends who might mean much in one's life.

The realization that there are people in life who will pose as friends, because in some way an individual is useful to them, and who will drop him as soon as the novelty wears off and they meet another who seems for the moment more attractive or useful, is one that comes to many nurses as one of the bitter experiences of life; but it is by such experience that one learns to be cautious in the choice of one's friends, and to be chary about becoming too intimate with those whose character and loyalty are open to question. Under the influence of so-called friends, a nurse is often led into going to places the character of which is open to question, and to doing unwise things which her own judgment condemns, and which lessens the confidence that others repose in her. This constitutes one of the commonest perils of friendship.

What is a Friend?—What are the chief things which a friend may rightly expect of us?

It is never desirable for a nurse to restrict her circle of friends to nurses or other workers in the same field. She needs the stimulus of new lines of thought. She needs a point of contact with people, both men and women, who are not of the world of sickness, who do not look out on life and its problems through the windows of a hospital, or of a sick-room, or of a doctor's office.

The elements of friendship are hard to analyze, but one thing is certain, that real friendship is always unselfish. It will not prevent one from maintaining a kindly interest in other workers, and kindly pleasant relations with other friends.

For a nurse in training her most wholesome friendships will usually be made with those of her own class. Close friendships between pupil nurses and head nurses are rarely conducive to the best interests of the school. When such a friendship develops, charges of favoritism are frequently made, and the feeling that favoritism exists, reacts adversely both on the pupil and head nurse.

Similarly, it is seldom an unmixed blessing to find senior nurses choosing their closest friends from among the probationers or juniors. It is hard to keep one's affections always within the safest limits, yet it is just as well to know that friendship has its dangers, and to guard against these dangers when possible.

Will a Real Friendship ever Lead an Individual to do Wrong?—Is it possible to love the friend, and yet, at times, hate, or refuse to uphold the friend's actions? We know that all sorts of crimes are excused under the plea of "shielding a friend" and nurses will often have to meet the question as to how far one's duty to one's friend extends.

A nurse in her second year was dismissed because of her entanglement with one of the orderlies. In her junior year she had been severely reprimanded and warned because of a violent flirtation which developed between her and one of the porters. It was known that she was meeting the orderly secretly outside the hospital, and there were numerous evidences of unprofessional relations while both were on night duty. Finally the climax came and both she and the orderly were dismissed. The dismissed nurse wrote to her closest friend asking her to persuade the members of her class to sign a petition that she be reinstated as a member of the school? What is the friend's duty in this matter?

Suggested Subject for Written Work.—Prepare a short paper, giving your idea as to how a nurse in training may wisely plan to spend a two week's summer vacation, so that she may get the best possible results in renewed health and enthusiasm.

FOR DISCUSSION OR REVIEW

1. To what extent is a nurse's health while in a hospital in her own keeping?
2. What suggestions would you give to a nurse who wished to keep at her maximum health while in training?
3. Make a list of the rules of health which you have seen nurses violate since your entrance to the school.
4. Mention some causes of overstrain in nurses in the early months of training.

5. What is the effect of worry on the digestion, on the power to sleep, on the general health?

6. When worry seems to be settling into a habit, what can or should an individual do to combat it?

7. What is the best antidote for worry that has thus far been discovered?

8. Prepare a synopsis of the suggestions in this chapter on "How to be an optimist."

9. What additions would you make to the health laws mentioned in this chapter?

10. Mention several ways in which you have observed that nurses do not use good judgment in regard to recreation.

11. In the matter of recreation in off-duty periods, what three things would you suggest that a nurse try to secure; what three things try to avoid?

12. Which do you think is most likely to result in health failure—hard, but congenial work, or worry? Give reasons for your answer.

13. How many close true friends is an individual likely to have at one time?

14. Mention some things which a nurse must do if she desires to have a circle of congenial friends.

15. What are some of the perils of friendship in hospital life, and later on?

16. Give several reasons why a nurse needs to cultivate friendships among people who are not of the hospital household or in any way connected with the world of sickness.

17. Will a true friend ever lead a nurse into wrong-doing?

CHAPTER XIX

Ethical Standards for Head Nurses

The head nurse's position is one of increasing importance in hospital and nursing life. She comes into closer contact with physicians, patients and pupil nurses than it is possible for a principal or superintendent to come, and the tone and atmosphere of the ward or department is determined to a considerable extent by her standards of conduct and duty, and by her manner and temperament. The nurse who has proven successful as a head nurse of a department will find many other doors of opportunity awaiting her. The position is an important part of the preparation which many superintendents and principals have had for their work. It offers the young graduate opportunities of no mean order to secure executive experience.

Thus far little attempt has been made to provide a special course for head nurses in hospitals that would help them to better understand their place in the whole plan of the hospital activities, but this no doubt will be reached in time. There is not and probably there never can be a fixed code of ethics for her. She will always have to learn much by experience and observation; but there are certain fundamental principles in ethics which pertain especially to the head nurse—principles which affect so vitally the harmony and tone and comfort of the whole institution that some time may wisely be spent in considering them.

The Head Nurse's Efficiency Record.—In a previous chapter reference was made to the efficiency record kept for pupil nurses, and the point was made that the pupil

GENERAL HOSPITAL

EFFICIENCY RECORD FOR HEAD NURSES

Name............	Position held.......	Vacation...........
Home address.....	Length of service...	Illness.............
Religion..........	Salary.............	Absences, reasons..

Personality:	Loyalty:
Courtesy..................	To Institution..............
Kindness..................	To Superintendent and principal....................
Enthusiasm................	To physicians..............
Ability to inspire these......	Respect for authority.........
Executive ability............	Observance of rules...........
Initiative................	Manner to subordinates
System..................	" " Patients........
Organizing powers..........	Professional manner toward:
General control...........	Internes..................
Progressiveness:	Visiting physicians..........
Study of nursing literature...	Visitors..................
Current literature.........	Temperament...............
Notetaking on newer methods...............	Judgment..................
Originality in plans of work.	Tact and resourcefulness.......
Improvements made or suggested...............	Economy..................
Ambition to excel..........	Effectiveness in carrying responsibility...............
Lack of................	
Teaching qualities:	
Theoretical work...........	
Practical work............	
Example to pupils:	
Good......Bad.........	
General interest in work of school................	

made these records herself—the principal of the school wrote down for future reference the record made in the everyday work. This is true also of head nurses and their records. What should an efficiency record for a head nurse contain? Opinions will differ on this point, but the specimen record will serve as an illustration for this chapter.

It will be seen from the foregoing form of record that there is abundant scope for the best powers of a graduate nurse in filling well such a position. The old conception of the head nurse's work was that of a supervisor whose duty it was to see that orders were carried out and the patients well cared for—and to this limited conception many aspirants for head nurse positions still tenaciously cling, seeing nothing beyond the getting of routine work done. The new conception which is being forced on nurses by the demands of the age is that she is not only a supervisor and executive, but a *teacher* who has exceptional opportunities to teach much of practical value which will never be taught, unless she measures up to her opportunity. While this new conception makes more demands on the nurse it has in it great possibilities for the development of the head nurse's own powers.

The Head Nurse's Example.—It is said of Emerson that he once wrote a young girl in whom he was much interested that he cared little concerning the name of the school which she had decided to attend, but that he cared much about the teachers under whose direction she worked and studied. A prominent educator, in speaking of the character of the instructors of the youth of our land, said that if he had his way there would be over the door of every school in the land a motto embodying this sentiment: "No teacher shall be employed in this school, whose character we would not desire reproduced, or whose example we would not wish every child in the land to copy." There are many in the hospital and training school field who have equally high standards for head nurses in hospital schools. Certainly the head nurse should be satisfied with nothing but the highest standard of life and conduct for herself. Next to experience the best of all teachers for nurses as well as other pupils is a good example. *No head nurse can hope to attain to the best standards for her class unless she is willing to sacrifice.* This is where many nurses fail when the crucial test comes.

Granted that a head nurse sincerely desires to become the best sort of example to pupils and to measure up as nearly as possible to the opportunities which her position affords her, what are some of the things which she should do and avoid doing?

The quality of fairness is one which every successful head nurse should try to possess. It must be one of the foundation stones in her system of management in her department, to be lived up to whether it be easy or difficult. This rule of fairness must extend throughout her whole department—to patients, to pupils, to doctors, to all who are associated with her. It is but natural to like some patients, doctors or pupils better than others, but justice should keep an executive from allowing her likes and dislikes to influence her management. Favoritism in any way usually leads to trouble.

Favoritism in regard to doctors frequently develops insiduously. A certain doctor has numerous patients in the hospital, and is anxious for favors to be shown to them. He perhaps boasts to his patients that he can secure such favors. It gives the patient the impression that he stands higher in the esteem of the hospital than his medical associates. He perhaps begins by flattering the young head nurse, and suggests some special reason why she should give special attention to one of his patients. She tries to do this, and later he presents a box of candy which, he remarks, is for "favors shown." The practice of showing favors grows. The other doctors, in course of time, learn that this certain doctor can get "anything he wants for his patients," and gradually, ripples of dissatisfaction arise which react adversely on the hospital, and the blame for which is often laid on the superintendent or principal who are unconscious of the real conditions which exist.

The fine art of finding fault pleasantly is one which every head nurse must cultivate. Much of her work must of necessity consist of correction or reproof, and the way in which this is done will have much to do with the good-feeling and harmony of the school. No really successful head nurse will allow herself to administer reproofs in the presence of others. This is always resented. To be able to administer rebuke without arousing antagonism is a quality which must be given diligent cultivation, and there is plenty of opportunity to practise this particular virtue.

Loyalty.—The head nurse who would inspire loyalty in pupils must herself be loyal. We like to think of some of the head nurses whom we have known who were towers of strength to the institution of which they were a part. Everything which affected its interest was to them a matter of deep concern. Without meddling in other departments, they frequently had knowledge of matters which affected the institution adversely, and a quiet word was spoken to the principal or superintendent. To the nurses they were never familiar yet never unapproachable. Every pupil felt that when she had personal matters of real importance under consideration she could talk them over with the head nurse, sure of her sympathy and wise counsel, and sure that her confidence would be respected. Loyalty is such a big intangible thing that it is difficult to go into details about it, but the following quotation from one of the well-known philosophers of this age, is worthy of consideration. Elbert Hubbard's voice was stilled when the Lusitania sank, but he left behind many bits of practical wisdom of which this on loyalty is one. He said:

"If you work for a man, in Heaven's name work for him. If he pays wages that supply you your bread and butter, work for him, speak well of him, stand by him, and by the institution which he represents. I think if I worked for a man I would work for him. I would not work for him part of his time, but all of his time. I would give him hearty, undivided service or none. If put to the pinch, an ounce of loyalty is worth a pound of cleverness.

"If you must vilify, condemn, and eternally disparage, why resign your position, and when you are outside criticize and "knock" to your heart's content. But, I pray you, so long as you are a part of an institution, do not condemn it. Not that you will injure the institution—not that—but when you disparage the concern of which you are a part, you disparage yourself."

Was Elbert Hubbard right or wrong in his conception of the duty of any individual who is a part of an institution? Show how his advice if followed would be helpful to an institution, and also to the individuals employed in it.

Appreciation of work well done and of general improvement is an important habit, for a head nurse to cultivate. There are but few individuals who will keep up sustained effort to improve, if nobody cares or seems to notice. Careless thinking and practice in pupils can often be traced to lack of appreciation of their best efforts.

Seeing beneath the surface is another quality which head nurses need to develop. Minor failures and errors are to be expected of pupil nurses, and while they are not to be overlooked, it is necessary that an effort be made to look beneath the surface and appreciate the spirit which was behind the failure. It takes no special amount of genius or skill to find fault. It does take skill to know when it is wise to overlook a failure, or how best to call attention to it, so that it will not occur again. It takes skill to be able to give constructive suggestions that will help to correct known faults.

Progressiveness and ambition are always found in the successful head nurse. She is constantly looking about for methods which will add to the efficiency of her department, yet careful before introducing them to talk them over with the principal. This latter point needs special emphasis because much trouble is caused by head nurses trying to institute new methods or teach them to nurses, while the head nurse in the next department to which the nurses go may disparage the method and refuse to have it used. There must be harmony in methods or much confusion is sure to result.

A superintendent's policy regarding head nurses was once stated to the author in this way. He said: "I like to hold out to our graduates the opportunity of head nurse positions in our hospital, but I have about decided to insist on every graduate securing at least six months in one or more institutions, before she begins her work with us. I have found that graduates who have done this, have brought back to us a freshness and enthusiasm that is worth much. They have gotten rid of the self-complacent spirit so common among nurses; and are able to bring to us many little practical points which have proven of great value to us. They find that other hospitals have difficulties quite as hard to meet as any we have, and they are able to take a much broader view of their work."

What do you think of this superintendent's policy regarding head nurses? Show where it is wise or unwise.

The head nurse's point of view has much to do with the smooth running of the hospital machinery. To be successful she must be able to see, to some extent at least, the needs of the institution as a whole, and to adapt herself to those needs without grumbling or unwise comment on particular situations. Failure to do this is a sign of unfitness for the work, or for greater responsibilities. A pupil nurse fails to report for duty on account of illness or several unusually sick patients come into one department, while in another there may be very few seriously ill patients. The principal decides to take a nurse from the department where the work is lighter, and place her where she is more needed. This has to be done for the good of the service, and it should be accepted without comment or question just as a good soldier accepts his orders.

Should this spirit of hearty coöperation be lacking in an institution, what can be done to create it?

Is it possible for a head nurse whose energies have to be largely if not wholly confined to one department of a hospital, to appreciate the needs of the institution as a whole? How far does selfishness enter into this particular problem?

A certain head nurse makes no secret of the fact that she wishes to secure a position as principal of a training school. She seems singularly lacking in resourcefulness and managing ability. For example, should a nurse be reported as ill, the head nurse invariably telephones the principal's office asking for another nurse to be sent to take the place of the one who is ill. It seems to never occur to her that she should try to adjust her plans so as to tide over the emergency without extra help. She acts as if she imagined that the principal kept nurses sitting in rows in her office ready at once to be sent to her relief.

Should such a head nurse expect a hospital to recommend her for the position she desired? What other qualities than those mentioned does she seem to lack?

Professional Conduct.—What is it? Try to write down a definition which would convey to the uninitiated the phases of conduct the term is intended to cover. It is far too wide a subject to be fully discussed here, but one or two phases of it which especially concern the discipline of the school may be considered. An illustration will perhaps explain more clearly one of the points that needs to be emphasized by the head nurse who desires to be counted successful, and who wishes to secure some position of greater responsibility.

Dr. B., a young practitioner, makes frequent visits to a hospital in which graduate nurses are in charge of departments. There are also always a number of graduate nurses on special duty. Dr. B. is genial and pleasant. His patients are not so numerous but that he has plenty of time to waste. Wherever he goes in the hospital, the head nurses and graduates on special duty gather about him for a "jolly good time." "He is so jolly" they say. All sorts of frivolous subjects are discussed. Jokes and stories are interchanged. The patients are disturbed by the talking and laughter. The special duty nurses should be with their patients. The head nurse should be attending to her duties. Treatments are delayed or neglected. Patients' calls are unanswered; just complaints arise. The efficiency of the service is lowered—all because of thoughtless but unprofessional conduct. Should this condition be corrected? If so, who should do the correcting? Suggest ways and means to control this sort of situation.

The worst thing about this phase of unprofessional conduct is that it is apt to be contagious. Others are led into doing things which they would not think of doing, had they not seen some one else doing it. The example of the head nurse is perhaps followed in some such fashion as this. A pupil nurse begins to gossip with an interne when he comes to her ward. To do this she has to neglect her work, many times. Occasionally she may even telephone that he "is wanted" in her ward, when she has some particularly delectable bit of "fudge" or other confection to distribute—such things do sometimes happen in twentieth century hospitals. Other nurses follow the example of this nurse, and so the undesirable practice extends. Show how this practice affects hospital efficiency. How does it affect a nurse's ideals of conduct? How the tone of the school?

Another phase of unprofessional conduct is shown in lack of respect for authority shown by some nurses. No one is fitted to command who has not learned to obey without grumbling, or questioning. This was one of the principles laid down by Florence Nightingale, and the years that have passed have proven the soundness of her contention that a well-trained nurse—a nurse who is fitted for the responsibility of directing others—must observe rules made for the good of all and must respect the wishes of those in authority over her. No nurse who is really fitted for head nurse responsibility will wish or try to be "a law unto herself."

Teaching Qualities.—In the efficiency record for the head nurse occurs the item of "teaching qualities." This is a point at which many good head nurses seem singularly timid, and there is no one who has not faced a class of nurses for the first time, who cannot understand to some degree the feeling of hesitation about assuming this responsibility. It is one thing to have a certain kind of knowledge, and a different thing to impart it effectively. There is a current belief that the teaching instinct is born with an individual—in other words that teachers as well as nurses "are born, not made." To some extent this may be true, but it would surprise most people if they really knew how much of thought and study and effort the supposed "born teacher" had put forth to reach a stage of proficiency that even approached her own ideals of teaching. There is usually a vast difference between what the individual was by native endowment, and what she has become by the study of the art of imparting knowledge. We did not know that we could walk till we tried, and we cannot know whether or not we can teach until we have really tried.

What mental picture have you of a successful teacher of nurses?

How may a head nurse develop her latent teaching ability?

First among the teaching qualities which the head nurse should cultivate is how to utilize to the fullest extent the teaching opportunities of her ward or department, so that pupil nurses really get the benefit of the clinical material before them. She needs to study how to tie up the theoretical teaching which a nurse has received, to the ward work. A lesson in bacteriology that seemed very dry or uninteresting may be given a practical application that the nurse will never forget, by reference to some patient in the ward. And this holds true throughout the course.

The art of questioning occupies a most important place in teaching. In fact a well-known educator has said that "the success and efficiency of our teaching depends more on the skill and judgment with which we put questions than on any other single method used in theoretical teaching."

Mention several kinds of questions which may be used to advantage—also kinds of questions which should be avoided.

What are the elements of a good answer?

Repetition is everywhere an important element in successful teaching. There is so much in hospital life to distract that few lessons are learned by "once telling." By degrees we learn that the pupil is not always to blame because she did not retain the thing we thought we had taught her. Perhaps we ourselves did not make the point quite clear, and did not properly emphasize it.

Patience with the slow pupil is another quality which head nurses need to cultivate. What methods have you seen used, or would you recommend to help the nurse who is slow in getting through her tasks, if she is otherwise qualified for nursing responsibilities?

These are just a few of the points which a nurse who aspires to become a really successful head nurse needs to consider—one who earnestly desires to do her duty and fill her place in the best manner possible.

Suggested Subject for Written Work.—Prepare a description of the head nurse whom you have met who most nearly approached your ideal. Tell what qualities you most admired in her.

FOR DISCUSSION OR REVIEW

1. Show why the head nurse is such an important factor in hospital life.

2. Explain what is meant by "professional conduct" in a nurse.

3. Tell why you think nursing is a profession and not a trade.

4. Why does the public seem to expect higher standards of conduct from professional people than from tradespeople?

5. Give some examples of conduct in institutional nurses that you considered unprofessional conduct.

6. To what extent do you consider it permissible in nurses to discuss affairs relating to the hospital, its working staff, or the patients, with their personal friends or the people of their own family?

7. If a nurse transgressed this rule, would you consider that she had been guilty of "unprofessional conduct?"

8. What is loyalty? Of what value to a nurse is a reputation for loyalty?

9. If a nurse is lacking in ambition to measure up to the responsibilities or demands of a position what can be done to make her a success?

10. What is the difference between "holding a position" and "filling a position?"

11. Should a nurse expect to hold a position which she does not try to fill wisely and well?

12. What is the difference between the old conception of a head nurse's responsibility and the new, as mentioned in this chapter? Which offers the greater possibilities of development to the nurse herself?

SECTION III

CHAPTER XX

After Graduation

What shall I do after graduation? How and where shall I use the training I have acquired? These are questions that press insistently on a nurse during her final year of training. Where does duty lie, when one ventures beyond the training school? What should the individual nurse's aim be as she leaves the school?

It is well for a nurse to have a dual aim in view, an immediate or present aim and an ultimate aim, something ahead to strive to reach. It is not well for her to be too positive at first about what she will or will not do. The path of duty is rarely clearly marked out very far ahead. We advance step by step. We live one day at a time. We do not need to see tomorrow's duty. We do not know what opportunity is going to offer us. We do know that experience as an independent worker is necessary, and a valuable asset. The opportunity most coveted will rarely be waiting for a nurse as she leaves the school, but the lesser opportunity which may prove the first step toward it will probably present itself in due time.

The most important thing for a nurse to examine herself in, when she faces the wide field of nursing, is regarding her own attitude of mind toward nursing, her own ideals of service. Is she conscious of a sincere desire to be broadly helpful in her own sphere, to go where she is needed most, to play well her part in the drama of life? Does she recognize any obligations of service to humanity

THE HIPPOCRATIC OATH*

"You do solemnly swear, each one by whatever she holds most sacred—

1. "That you will be loyal to the physicians under whom you shall serve, as a good soldier is loyal to his officers;

2. "That you will be just and generous to all worthy members of your profession, aiding them when it shall be in your power so to do;

3. "That you will lead your lives and practise your profession in uprightness and honor;

4. "That into whatsoever house you enter, it shall be for the good of the sick to the utmost of your power, and that you will hold yourselves aloof from all temptation;

5. "That whatsoever you shall see or hear of the lives of men and women, whether they be your patients or members of their households, you will keep inviolably secret, whether you are in other households or among your own friends.

"If you accept these obligations, let each one bow the head in sign of acquiescence.

"And now, if you shall be true to your word, may prosperity and good repute be ever yours; the opposite, if you shall prove yourselves forsworn."

* Note.—This pledge is a modification of the Hippocratic Oath used by some medical schools and, so far as is known, was first used in the New York City Training School for Nurses.

because of the opportunity which has been hers to become a skilled workman? Has she adopted for herself any guiding principles which, if followed, will help her to make the most of life and yield the greatest possible sum of happiness to herself and others?

If a nurse desires a life that is abundant, rich, and satisfying, yielding a full measure of happiness, she will find it through service, and in no other way. The law of happiness is based on social service, or service to society, service to others. Happiness comes to us indirectly, and refuses to come if sought as an end in itself. There can be no service in the real sense of the term without some degree of sacrifice, though the sacrifice is usually unconscious and its chief element is self-forgetfulness.

Guiding Ethical Principles.—"For whosoever will save his life shall lose it; and whosoever will lose his life for my sake shall find it." "All things whatsoever ye would that men should do to you, do ye even so to them." These two guiding principles, if applied by every nurse in her own life, will solve many of the perplexing questions that beset the young nurse. The nursing body will be lifted to a higher level only as the life of the individual nurse is improved, and only as she brings herself into conformity with these great laws of human welfare.

Had Florence Nightingale sought her own happiness and convenience, had she planned for herself a life of ease, she would never have carved for herself a niche in the most enduring of all temples of fame—the hearts of the people.

Had Jane Addams lost sight of the two great guiding principles of life just quoted, she would never have been known as one of the greatest women of her time. Thus examples might be quoted indefinitely which go to prove the enduring truths expressed, truths which are as vital today as when first uttered, fundamental truths which have but begun to do their work, truths which need to be personally applied by every nurse.

Are your ideals of service copied from some other nurse who may be far from successful in the best sense of the word, or are they the ideals of service given by the Great Teacher?

To what extent is an individual responsible for the actions of others?

How does a private nurse act who puts self first in her plans and purposes?

How does putting self first affect the comfort and well-being of an institutional worker and the institution? What effect is it likely to have on real success as a nurse?

What is the power of a vision?

What is the best way for a nurse to set about making her dreams of service come true?

How should success be measured in a nurse's life?

What had a vision of the world's needs to do with Florence Nightingale's work? How did she set about making her dreams a reality?

What are your highest ideals? What is involved in being loyal to those ideals?

The Value of a Life Purpose.—The most practical people do more or less dreaming about the things they are going to make happen, or at least are going to try to make happen. Before effective action there must come thinking, and thinking till a purpose is reached. Every nurse has opportunities to make the world better if she cares to use them. They are everywhere, and great movements often begin with the doing of some concrete thing that was badly needing to be done at the moment.

The life story of Jacob Riis as told in "The Making of an American" is an apt illustration of the power of a vision and the force of a life purpose in our own day. He died in 1913, but before he died he dreamed dreams of a better New York, and made his dreams come true in large measure. He struggled with poverty, loneliness, the disadvantages of having to acquire a new language in the land of his adoption, but the power of a vision of better conditions which he could help bring about held him steady in times of despondency. He was far too busy in his early years in this country trying to keep himself and family clothed and fed to plan any very big programs of constructive philanthropy, but he saw the things that were not right, and persistently told of them by tongue and pen and kodak. He presented not problems, but *people who needed to be helped* to decent living conditions. *He set himself the task of making people see*—a big task that can be worked at anywhere. He set up new standards of life for the poor, and did what he could to have those standards accepted. It is a long story, but wonderfully captivating. It has many lessons for nurses.

The established order of things sometimes has to be upset before much progress can be made. There are conditions that are not right in regard to nursing which should be worked at till better conditions are assured. In the private nursing field especially, nurses are most unequally distributed—patients who sadly need their skill are unable to secure it; nurses who seriously need work are held back from accepting calls to nurse where their help is sorely needed. To illustrate: A widow who was left with a little girl of five, and dependent on her own efforts for a living for both, was advised by her family doctor to "take up nursing" as a practical nurse, promising that he and a few of his medical associates would keep her busy. His first call on her was to care for a maternity patient, which she did for two weeks—the only experience she had had in nursing outside of her own family. The morning after she returned from her first case, a doctor called on her to go to a patient of his whom he said had some "stomach trouble." She went and found a very serious case of gastric ulcer, with hemorrhages, persistent vomiting, severe pain, and with a serious heart complication besides. There were two little children in the home. The husband had to keep at work to earn their daily bread. This practical nurse was ordered to feed the patient entirely by rectum, and on the doctor's next visit all medicine by mouth was stopped and ordered to be given by hypodermic. The practical nurse, after struggling with the case for two days, filled with dread every moment that the patient would die after one of the severe vomiting attacks, gave up the case and went home, saying to the family that a trained nurse was needed. They begged her to stay—the doctor did the same—the family said they were unable to pay the price for a trained nurse and a servant to do the work besides, but she refused to remain longer in charge of such a serious case. Did she do right? What should have been done? This kind of problem could be duplicated hundreds of times every year in every community. What should be the attitude of the young graduate toward this sort of problem? Can she do anything to change the existing order of things? What attitude would Florence Nightingale have taken toward such cases? What can or should one nurse do toward meeting the responsibility presented in this problem?

Some one has said that "Every great advance in science has had as its beginning and first cause a new point of view. Every epoch-making discovery has implied a way of looking at things different from that which has previously prevailed. Civilization advances as new points of view prevail. The great lights in the world's history give us new points of view."* The importance of getting a correct viewpoint, one which will enable her to see the needs of the world and what the individual nurse could or should do to meet them, cannot be too strongly emphasized.

Industry.—Next in importance to getting the right viewpoint and securing right guiding principles of conduct and life is that of cultivating right habits. When one leaves the training school and new conditions have to be met, habits are more or less disturbed and discipline is relaxed. This is a time in which a nurse especially needs to be on her guard, lest the good habits she has formed slip away and bad habits take their place.

One of the essentials to success in any branch of nursing is industry—willingness to work. It makes little difference how capable and skilled a nurse may have become during her training, if she is not willing to work; if she is continually looking out for the easiest cases and places and refusing those which would probably mean serious or hard work, she can never be a successful nurse. Quite frequently a nurse who is a habitual shirker may be able to get through a training school because someone constantly supervised her and kept her up to the mark, but when she becomes an independent worker, her habitually lazy habits reassert themselves. This type of nurse does more to create prejudice against trained nurses than any other type. A train of complaints follow such nurses wherever they go. They are unaccommodating in private homes, and always fearful lest they will be

* Richard T. Ely, in Social Law of Service.

imposed on by being asked to do something which is not directly connected with the patient. They apply for hospital positions and often secure them, but fail to measure up to the opportunity that is theirs. They make frequent changes, and usually have nothing good to say of those who have employed them. Their habitual unwillingness to work shows up more plainly in private homes than anywhere else, for under those conditions there is no one whose duty it is to keep them up to the mark.

A young graduate of a large training school when filling out an application for a place on the school registry stated that she would not go to the country; would not do night work; would not nurse nervous or mental patients; would not take tuberculosis cases or the acute contagious diseases; would not nurse obstetrical patients or children. In what qualities essential for success in nursing was this nurse lacking? Who was responsible for this lack, the nurse or her training school? What sort of service might reasonably be expected of such a nurse on the cases to which she agreed to go?

What general results would follow so far as the nursing body is concerned if all graduate nurses went out with the spirit shown by this nurse and followed her example? How would the welfare of the sick be affected? What should be the attitude of other graduates of the same school toward this nurse? Can they do anything to change her attitude?

Adaptability.—Closely related to industry is the quality of adaptability, and both of them have their roots in unselfishness. Lack of adaptability does not always mean selfishness pure and simple, but there is nearly always an element of selfishness in it. The nurse who lacks adaptability "fusses" when she cannot have her own way, is unable to see a situation from the viewpoint of others, is unable or unwilling to concede to others the rights which she demands for herself. Her own convenience and comfort are usually uppermost in her mind, though she would be the last to admit it.

To a certain extent lack of adaptability may be due to training, but not wholly. No nurse is wholly the product of her school; she can correct defects in character if she really desires to. The chief difficulty lies in the unwillingness to recognize her own defects and limitations or the reasons for her failures. She too frequently suffers from what Florence Nightingale termed "the vice of self-sufficiency." She wants people who employ her to bend to her ways. She does not make a real effort to "fit into" the varying situations in which she finds herself, so there is constant friction. She may be a capable nurse but "hard to get along with." She does not realize that "pleasing the patient" is one of the most important elements in her success as an independent worker. In the hospital it is always a detriment to a nurse if it can be said of her: "Her patients do not like her;" in private nursing it is always a calamity.

A nurse trained in a large city hospital enters the private nursing field. She had practically always done her work in a large ward. Her patients have been of the very poorest class. She can manage her share of the nursing in a large ward well, but has never during her training had the time to devote herself to caring for but one patient at a time. Her patients did not demand a lot of fussy attention, and had to be satisfied with having their actual needs attended to. How is this nurse to so change her habits that she will be a successful nurse to one private patient in her home surrounded by family and friends? What are the chief things against which she must guard? What suggestions would you offer such a nurse that might be helpful to her in meeting the difficulties of such a situation in a home in which the patient was a young wife who had been accustomed to the refinements and luxuries of life?

Making a good first impression is important whatever line of nursing may be chosen. It is especially important for the private nurse. The patients who furnish the demand for her services are ill, and usually abnormally sensitive in mind and body; their friends and relatives are, frequently, even more sensitive than the patient himself. Impressions made at such times are more vivid than usual. Many invalids, especially those of a nervous type, are unusually influenced by certain personalities; they often take violent likes or dislikes without knowing why. They are "easily rubbed the wrong way"—easily irritated. Very often, where a nurse makes a wrong impression at the start, the doctor disposes of the problem by promptly sending the nurse away. He refuses to add to the physical strain which his patient has to endure, the unnecessary mental strain of having either to conquer a dislike or endure it. By failing to make the right impression in such a case, the nurse creates a prejudice against herself which will react adversely on her where future calls are concerned. Granted that a nurse earnestly desires to make a good impression, how shall she manage it? It is well to remember that first impressions are gained from superficial things, from appearances, largely from dress and manner. A nurse who is dressed like a walking fashion plate, with an elaborate style of hairdressing or much jewelry, is apt to give the impression that she is likely to be more interested in her personal appearance than in her work or the care of the patient. Neatness in dress and a sense of the fitness of things is expected of her.

A nurse's manner reflects to a degree her inner qualities. Two things which go far toward making a good impression are a sincere interest in the patient to be served, not a feigned interest or a "case" interest, and a spirit of genuine kindness that finds its expression in numerous indefinable ways. A nurse who is genuinely kind will find that that virtue covers up a multitude of other defects.

"Another important constituent of a good impression is self-confidence. This must be guarded that it shall not become conceit, which always offends and antagonizes. This quality is a necessary one. If you have not a good opinion of yourself, how are you going to impress others that you are worthy of their good opinion? If you are not reasonably sure that you can do a thing, how are you to get a chance to do it? If you seem not to be mistress of the situation, how are you going to make people willing to let you undertake their affairs? A man who respects himself is bound to be respected. A woman who is willing and knows that she can do good work is likely to be given an opportunity to do it."

Practically all that has been said about the value of first impressions to the private nurse applies with equal force to institutional nursing and to other lines of work. The wearing of much jewelry and a lingerie blouse cut indecently low in the neck has prevented a nurse from securing a coveted position in an institution. The superintendent decided that the jewelry was unnecessary for nurses and indicated personal vanity, and the indecently low-cut blouse suggested that its wearer would not be a good example to pupil nurses.

The failure to keep an appointment made for a certain hour has often settled the question of the desirability of a nurse for some desired position. She was unbusinesslike and was likely to fail in various other directions.

The best positions come to those who are willing to pay the price of prolonged study and training. As a rule, such positions require women of sterling character and a wholesome ambition to excel in their chosen line. Success is not a matter of chance.

The Carrying of Responsibility.—The ease and effectiveness with which a nurse is able to assume responsibility determines her value in large measure. This fact cannot be too strongly emphasized. The nurse who habitually shirks responsibility, or fails to measure up to it, is not worth as much in dollars and cents to an institution, organization, or family as the nurse who quietly takes on burdens of responsibility and faithfully carries them. A nurse determines her own value very soon by her attitude toward responsibility, and toward human needs in home, hospital, or elsewhere.

Earnest effort to measure up to the responsibilities that come all along the way, combined with industry and adaptability, will do more to pave the way to better positions with greater responsibilities than any other thing. It is as true today as ever it was that he who has been faithful in a few things, in lesser responsibilities, is the one who is going to be given greater responsibilities. Friends may recommend and help to secure a desired position for a nurse, but it rests with herself whether she fills the position satisfactorily. Friends cannot make good her character deficiencies. Training alone will not bring success.

The world cares but little how many degrees a nurse has, or how many diplomas. These serve as certificates of a certain amount of preparatory attainment, but they will not save the unfit from failure. The world that is represented in the great wide field now open to nurses is looking always for the nurse who has shown herself capable of bearing real burdens, of carrying responsibilities, of exercising the right influence on others, of doing things, of directing others, of getting results. A reputation for measuring up to responsibilities wherever her work has called her is worth more to the average nurse than a university degree. The latter is a good thing to have, but unless a nurse manifests the three qualities named—industry, adaptability, and the ability to easily and effectively assume responsibility—her university degree will not make her a success in any line of nursing endeavor.

Suggested Subject for Written Work.—How may a nurse cultivate the quality of seeing a given situation from the viewpoint of those who employ her?

QUESTIONS FOR DISCUSSION OR REVIEW

1. How much does one's mental attitude toward nursing have to do in influencing the success of any worker?
2. Outline what you consider is the right mental attitude of the nurse at graduation toward the needs of the world and the problems that confront her.
3. Is it possible for a nurse to really be true to section 5 of the pledge found on page 220? How many nurses do you know who have violated that pledge? Is it more difficult to keep than the other clauses in the pledge? If so, why?
4. Mention three important qualities for a nurse to possess who desires to be entrusted with large responsibilities.
5. What do you understand by adaptability and how is it cultivated? Show why it is important in a nurse's success.
6. How is a nurse who is not adaptable liable to act in a private home?

7. How far is a nurse to be blamed for her lack of adaptability? Could she overcome it if she desired to?

8. How does a nurse show while in a training school that she is fitted for a position of responsibility?

9. Give some suggestions to a nurse who desires to make a good first impression.

10. Mention two qualities which help a nurse to make a good impression.

CHAPTER XXI

The Wide Field

The nursing field, into which the young graduate enters, widens from year to year, as new ways are discovered of bringing the skill and training of a nurse to bear on the needs of the world. From the training school one may find over twenty different lines radiating, each leading to a somewhat different kind of service in which nurses may engage.

Vocations for Nurses.—In a training-school announcement, recently received, the following list of "vocations" appears:

Superintendent of hospital.
Assistant superintendent of hospital.
Principal of training school.
Assistant principal of training school.
Head nurses of departments.
Instructors in training schools.
Hospital social service nurse.
Dietitian.
Hospital office assistant.
Anesthetist.
Resident nurse in schools and colleges.
Private duty nurse.
Army and Navy nurse.
Red Cross nurse.
Rural nursing service.
District nurse.
Office nurse.
School nurse.

Social welfare workers.
Foreign missionary workers.
Tuberculosis nurse.
Infant welfare nurse.
Almshouse nurse.
Sanitary inspectors.
Department store nurse.

If the number of vocations which mean opportunity for service seems bewildering, the problem of choice may be simplified if one remembers that the great majority of nurses will naturally come in one of the three great divisions of nursing:

Institutional work.
Private nursing in homes.
Visiting nursing and public health work.

The institutional field each year demands more and more workers, as higher standards of service in institutional work and additional buildings create the demand. Hospitals are living growing things, constantly enlarging, and each year new institutions come into existence. The regular hours, freedom from outside expenses, generally good accommodation, and the spirit of comradeship in service found in hospitals all combine to make this form of nursing attractive. Where a few years ago one found one or two paid graduate workers in a hospital, one may today find ten or more in the same institution.

The great variety of positions in institutional work calls for a variety of talent. At the door of many hospitals one finds a nurse who serves as an admitting officer—receiving patients, meeting their friends, and answering the multitude of questions that come to one in such a position. What temperament and qualifications should a nurse have for such a position?

In another, one may find a nurse in charge of the bookkeeping and clerical work with other assistants provided.

In another, one finds a nurse in charge of the dietary department and also acting as matron of the nurse's home, capable assistants being provided who work under her direction.

In another, one finds a nurse who has special qualifications as a teacher, visiting several hospitals weekly as instructor in certain subjects.

In another, one finds a nurse in charge of the nurse's home—having the responsibility of managing about their uniforms, arranging for social events for them, caring for sick nurses not ill enough to be in the hospital, serving as housemother, and with the office of assistant to the principal.

In another hospital one finds not one, but several nurses regularly employed as anesthetists.

A hospital starts a social service department with one nurse, and a little later it gives her one or two or more assistants, as the work grows, and results are seen that justify the expense.

In another institution one finds a nurse in charge of the entire instruction of probationers, carrying one class at a time through for perhaps two, three, or six months, and then admitting another. She specializes in this kind of work.

The increase in surgical work that is going on all over the country is requiring an army of skilled operating room nurses, and the demand for this class of worker grows each year.

Dispensary work is becoming every year a more important part of the hospital activities, and here and there dispensaries, independent of hospitals, are being started.

These all require one or more nurses for the most effective service, and to the nurse whose sympathies go out to the struggling poor, the dispensary offers a field of service of wonderful opportunity.

There is found, besides, a great increase in the number of head nurses and assistants to the principal or superintendent, and such work has many attractions.* One writing on the opportunities of the head nurse says: "The head nurse touches life on many sides. If she is interested in science, she may see in the ward the very latest application of it for the benefit of humanity. She may herself take part in the work, and by her knowledge and skill, help to make these new discoveries successful in the treatment of disease. She works side by side with physicians and surgeons whose work other men may cross continents to see. This is a constant stimulus to further study and effort.

"If it is sociology that fascinates her, the material for its study is all around her, for at one time or another all the great problems that social workers are grappling with, are encountered in the hospital ward.

"If it is humanity that calls to her, just elemental human nature with its comedy and pathos, its courage and its despair, its divinity, its degradation—all phases of it are revealed in the flashes of quaint humor, the patiently endured trouble, the little comedies and the stern tragedies of the hospital ward. Life never lacks interest here.

"Finally, if the maternal instinct is strong in her, and I believe that is the fundamental thing in all women who are good nurses, it may find a wholesome field for its expression in the care given to the sick, and in the very important part she takes in the professional education

* Marion G. Parsons.

of the young women who are to be the nurses of the future."

In the field of public health nursing, so-called, one finds a still greater development going on, and opportunity is provided for a wonderful variety of talent to find scope. Apart from the regularly organized forms of visiting nursing, now well understood, one finds nurses each year filling some new need. In one place one may find a nurse doing a sort of inspection duty in a neighborhood in which a number of cases of contagious disease exists. She not only instructs, advises and assists the families in which such diseases are present, but she is there to see that quarantine laws are observed.

Another nurse may be engaged solely in giving instruction to the school children of a city on how to prevent tuberculosis. She goes from school to school and tells her story, and even if the children sometimes call her "the spit nurse" they love her none the less.

Another nurse may be the only one of her class in a whole county—sent there by the State Board of Health to discover cases of tuberculosis and help to secure for them the help they need.

Nurses in a southern state have won the admiration of all who know of their work among the mountaineers, in fighting the spread of trachoma, and preventing many cases of blindness.

In other cities one finds "little mother's leagues" organized, with nurses in charge, giving instruction to school girls on how to care for their baby brothers and sisters.

As the infant welfare work becomes more fully organized, increased demands for nurses for this form of service will be made on those now in training. For the nurse who is able to give health lectures to mothers, and create interest in health matters in a community, there is a fine field of service.

The school nurse has made for herself a place of increasing importance in the country, while factories and department stores in greater numbers are finding need for a nurse's services.

The foreign field is calling loudly each year for nurses from America to come to take charge of hospitals and dispensaries in foreign fields where health work is so badly needed.

For many of these positions the nurse who is wise will take time to secure special training if she expects to render effective service. However complete a hospital training may be, it can constitute only the foundation for most of the forms of service mentioned.

Making a Choice.—In attempting to decide which one of these divisions to enter, it is well to take stock so far as one may, of one's own capabilities. To do good work in any of these fields requires that a nurse must have, besides her technical training, some enthusiasm, adaptability, and liking for the work. Occasionally one meets the unusual nurse, the nurse who apparently can follow any one of several different lines of work and appear to do well in all of them. Such nurses have probably acquired before and after coming to the training school a variety of experience and education along different lines, that serves to supplement their nurse training; and they have, besides, that important qualification known as executive ability. But the majority of nurses cannot do two or three kinds of work equally well. The difficulty with many nurses is that they become hopeless drifters, rarely staying at any one thing long enough to become really proficient, never being able to say of any one kind of work, "this is where I feel I can do the best work," or "I have found my work." Very often, a certain form of nursing has been idealized in the pupil nurse's mind. She sees it from a distance, and it appears to have a halo of glory around it. She may be honestly convinced that such work is the work of all others in the world for her. A bit of experience is then her greatest necessity. To illustrate: A young nurse full of ambition, after graduating from one hospital, immediately entered for further training in another. She was determined to leave nothing undone to secure the best preparation possible for her life's work. While taking the post-graduate course she became convinced that visiting nursing was the work she wanted above anything else. To "go about doing good" among the poor—could anything be more beautiful? It seemed from a distance to be the "ideal occupation" for her. Fortunately, the opportunity came to her soon after leaving the post-graduate school to substitute for a nurse who was doing visiting nursing under the auspices of a church organization. There was no one really to direct her work, or to give her a word of practical advice about it. A large part of the work consisted in visiting patients suffering from chronic disease, where her nursing duties were of the simplest sort. Long tedious hours were spent, in one or two cases, in combing long matted hair which had been badly neglected; at other times in giving baths to patients who protested against having them; other patients spent their money for stimulants and patent medicines that did not cure, but would not listen to her advice; much time was spent in carrying special delicacies to patients who were just as needy the next day, and would be till the end. Visiting nursing was then unorganized. Each center was an isolated unit. This nurse could not feel that she was part of a vast social movement for human betterment. She was simply an isolated worker doing tasks most of which she felt she could as easily have accomplished after a few months training. The halo around the work began to fade. When the time she had agreed to substitute had expired, she took an institutional position, became an efficient principal of a training school, and later superintendent of a hospital. She still "went about doing good" but in a hospital, for which work she was unusually well fitted. Other nurses have similarly idealized other lines of work. A nurse who had bubbled over with enthusiasm about "public health work" found her enthusiasm waning with the first prolonged period of rainy weather. She lacked imagination and stick-to-it-iveness.

There are disagreeable features in all branches of work, including nursing, and each has its compensations. There is such a thing, however, as "working against the grain," working in conditions which are singularly distasteful, and it is certain that one's best work will not be accomplished in such circumstances. There is an excess of nervous energy expended, where one is working against one's natural bent, where there is friction, and where one feels that there is not scope for the best use of one's powers, that in time reacts adversely on the health of the worker.

Two practical questions which a nurse may well ask herself in considering an occupation, therefore, are: Have I within myself the possibility of measuring up to the demands of this situation? Would I be happy in this particular line of work?

Making a Right Start.—There are several important ethical considerations which a nurse should especially try to keep in mind when she goes forth as an independent worker.

1. The public will judge trained nurses in general, by the conduct and spirit of individual nurses in their work.

2. A nurse's honor is at stake in many of the problems that will confront her.

3. In her dealings with the sick, or with the public, there are always at least two sides to every question that arises, and sometimes three or four sides. She must try to see these other sides.

A nurse's word should mean something if she ever hopes to attain to any position of trust. If she agrees to go to a certain place at a certain time, she should be there unless some accident befalls her, or she should notify in time those who are depending on her or expecting her that she cannot keep the engagement. To make such a reputation that people will say, "If Miss Blank said she'd be there, you can surely depend on her, she always keeps her word," is worth more to a nurse than she can readily estimate. If a nurse has no sense of honor, nothing within herself that will keep her from doing small contemptible things, the greatest benefit that she can confer on the nursing profession is to leave it.

A nurse who had graduated about four years before applied to her superintendent to help her to find a position. She had had a discouraging experience, and was both out of work and out of money. The only vacancy that the superintendent had to suggest at the time was with a visiting nurse association some distance away which was then in need of a worker. This was just the kind of work the nurse wanted, she said; so her application went at once. The nurse had committed no flagrant misdemeanors during her training; she had done "passably good" work, and the superintendent recommended her in a somewhat restrained non-committal manner. The nurse had had some few months of experience in visiting nursing, and it seemed as if she might give satisfaction if she really tried. On the strength of the superintendent's recommendation, the application was promptly accepted, and the day was set, about four weeks hence, on which she was to report for duty, to take the place of another nurse who was leaving to go to another position.

A few days before the date set for the nurse to begin service with the visiting nursing organization, the superintendent received a letter from a hospital to which this nurse had applied for a position as night superintendent, and shortly after another letter was received from a tuberculosis hospital to which the same nurse had applied for a position. It developed that *after the arrangements with the visiting nurse society had been made*, the nurse heard of the vacancy as night superintendent, and also saw an advertisement for nurses for the tuberculosis hospital. She could see no reason why the superintendent would not recommend her for any or all of them, though she had been under contract for weeks with another organization. There, apparently, was no question in her own mind as to her fitness to fill any of these positions. The obligations which she incurred when she accepted the position with the visiting nurse society were as nothing to her. It meant nothing to her that the visiting nurse work would be thrown into confusion, or that the welfare of the patients in the district that was to have been hers was to a degree dependent on her keeping her word. She thought the superintendent was most hard-hearted that she did not promptly write recommendations for her for all these positions, and as many more as she chose to apply for. In fact she thought only of her own side of the case. What ethical failures was this nurse guilty of? If this were an isolated case, it need not be given serious consideration, but it illustrates an ethical problem of no small magnitude, and one that is far too common. Engagements for service are accepted by nurses and broken with an indifference that is appalling. It is such nurses who drift aimlessly from place to place, never holding any position long enough to really make good, and often spending several months of the year idle.

How many positions may a nurse properly apply for at one time? If she has applied for more than one position, what course should she pursue when she finds one application accepted? Having accepted a position which proves distasteful to her, after a few weeks' experience, what should she do?

Depending on one's alma mater or on the hospital in which one has been trained, to keep one supplied with work, is a failing which is common in the nurse of today. Twenty years ago, or less, *no* nurse on graduation expected that she was to get her calls for nursing from the hospital in which she trained. Today one may find, in many places, that a whole class of nurses, instead of looking around to find out where their services are most needed, are inclined to settle down a few blocks from the hospital, to look to the hospital to send them special cases, to cast jealous eyes on the cases on which pupil nurses are given special nursing experience, and to find fault with the principal if she calls in some other nurse while they are idle. This unwholesome and dependent attitude of mind in regard to nursing, and to one's life work, is detrimental to the whole nursing body. It helps to keep nurses crowded in cities, while not far away there may be whole counties without a nurse.

The pioneer spirit is not dead in the nurses of today, but it is badly in need of better cultivation. It is true that most nurses will have to follow the pioneer, yet the spirit of the pioneer should be in every nurse. She should cultivate the courage to advance beyond the well-populated districts—confident that there is nothing in the "regions beyond" which a brave, healthy, well-trained nurse need fear to meet.

What is the pioneer spirit? What qualities do pioneers possess that many nurses of today seem to lack? What is the price of pioneering?

It depends on how far the pioneer spirit leads us, what the price is that we pay for it, and on how completely that spirit takes possession of us. If we study the life stories of the pioneers in nursing we will find that they seemed to scorn the cost—left it entirely out of consideration. If they had been afraid to venture outside of the city for fear they would not have hot and cold water always at hand, electric light, telephone service, someone to wait on them, etc., the world would never have heard much about them.

The Price of Pioneering is often Unpopularity.—There are those who will try to make the pioneer's plans seem ridiculous, who will raise obstacles, and who will hinder by their constant criticism of motives. The real pioneer must be able to go on in spite of these difficulties if he expects to accomplish anything worth while. Most great causes have at first been unpopular, and there will always be those who will urge the life of ease, and urge a nurse not to venture far away. How shall she cultivate the courage to go? How shall she discover where she is most needed?

The development of tuberculosis hospitals and nursing has put before the nurses of today a challenge which some nurses have met with wonderful bravery and success. Others have failed. The following form of ethical failure is not unusual. In a certain tuberculosis hospital, graduate nurses are employed for the general nursing of the patients. During the absence of the superintendent there was a certain amount of relaxation in regard to enforcement of rules, etc., and when the superintendent, on her return, endeavored to correct certain undesirable practices several graduate nurses promptly resigned, on a day's notice, and left the patients to the care of whomever the superintendent could pick up. This ethical failing of graduate nurses is not confined to tuberculosis hospitals, but can be readily illustrated in other institutions and places.

Even if a contract for service calls for no definite term of notice before leaving, should a nurse's sense of honor cause her to give ample notice? What considerations should guide her in cases of this kind? What can one nurse do to correct this condition?

The Need of Study.—Florence Nightingale nearly fifty years ago deplored the fact that nurses were more anxious for positions than they were to find out what the positions were desiring in them, and how near or how far they came from meeting the just expectations of those who employed them. To fill well some of the positions mentioned in this chapter requires that a nurse must be ready every year or two to take up some new kind of study. Visiting nurses need to be familiar with the methods of organized charity, "with new housing regulations which are made, to learn new facts about immigration, the best way of dealing with young girls whose surroundings make morality difficult, and to keep up with social as well as with medical progress." The nurse who neglects or refuses to study, soon falls behind, and finds it harder and harder to secure a satisfactory location. As long as she is in the work, a nurse should expect to be a student. She should invest in books and magazines as a mechanic does in tools, that she may keep abreast with the march of modern progress.

Suggested Subject for Written Work.—Prepare a short paper containing suggestions which might be helpful to a young nurse who was about to apply for an institutional position, things to do, things to avoid.

FOR DISCUSSION OR REVIEW

1. What is meant by the term "vocation?" In what sense does it differ from "occupation?"

2. Mention the three great divisions of the nursing field.

3. Outline briefly the difference in the qualities required for effective service in each of these fields.

4. State some important things which a nurse should consider before making a choice of any branch of nursing.

5. In applying for a position as chief surgical nurse in a distant city, what information may a nurse wisely and rightly ask for in regard to the place she is considering?

6. Make a list of the questions which a nurse may properly ask about a head nurse's position which she intends to apply for, also for a position as superintendent of a training school.

7. What is the value of experience in an executive position to a nurse? Would a nurse be wise at first to work for a comparatively small salary in order to secure experience? How should she rate the value of her services?

8. Mention the chief points on which a hospital board of managers is likely to wish to be informed regarding applicants for the following positions:

Superintendent of a hospital.

Principal of a training school.
Instructor of nurses.
Chief surgical nurse.

9. What suggestions would you give a nurse who wished to prepare herself for infant welfare work? What qualities should she possess?

10. Mention three books which you would advise a nurse who wanted a position as a school nurse to buy and study.

11. Give a list of books which might be helpful to a nurse who desired to secure employment as a social service worker in connection with a hospital.

12. Mention some qualities which a nurse in an executive position in a tuberculosis hospital should possess.

13. Write a short paper giving your idea of places in which pioneer work is needed in the United States? In Canada? Tell why you feel such work is needed and the kind of nurses needed to do it.

14. Give some reasons why nurses should not settle down close to the hospital in which they were trained. State some of the problems created by doing so.

15. Give some suggestions as to how the pioneer spirit may be developed in the nurse of today.

16. How many years after a nurse graduates should she need to send back to her training school for recommendations? To what extent should she depend on them to help her find her place in the wide field?

CHAPTER XXII

A Nurse and Her Money

A speaker in a public address to men, emphasized the point that the best index to a man's character was the use he made of the margin of his time—that part of it which was not devoted to work or sleep, or the actual necessities of life; another important indication of character mentioned was the way an individual spent the money he earned.

Would the application of these two tests, "How do you spend the margin of your time?" "What do you do with your money?" give any idea of character in the nurses you know?

The charge that nurses are unbusinesslike in their habits, inclined to extravagance, apt to live up to the extent of their incomes, is frequently made and with some degree of truth. Whether they are more improvident than other classes of workers, is an unsettled question.

The National Young Women's Christian Association recently appointed a committee on "thrift and efficiency." In a leaflet issued by that committee occur the following questions which nurses in common with other workers may wisely ask themselves:

FIVE PERTINENT QUESTIONS FOR A WOMAN EARNING A SALARY

1. How much have I earned all told in my life?
2. How much could I have saved if I had wanted to?
3. How much do I possess free and clear now?

4. How much of the difference between earnings and present possessions has been frittered away?

5. What am I going to do from this time on to secure my living expenses in sickness and in old age?

In considering one's duty, or in the study of ethics, it is certain that the right or the wise use of money should not be overlooked. It is also certain that it is easier to earn money than to spend it wisely, that the wise investment of the reward of one's own labor is one of the big problems of life. Whether one is considering the spending of one dollar or one thousand, the matter is an investment. To a great many young nurses, $25 a week seems a large sum, and in the first flush of elation over their wage-earning ability, they proceed to invest in various items of longed-for finery, and presently when work is slack they find themselves with no bank account, a very slim pocketbook, and expenses going steadily on.

Mention some reasons why a nurse should keep accurate account of income and expenditure from year to year.

Make a list of a model wardrobe for a private or institutional nurse, stating the approximate amount of each article, and the total cost.

If a private nurse's income amounts to $800 a year, what part of this amount should be devoted to each of following classes of expenses: Housing accommodation, food, clothing, recreation, books and magazines, health expenses, church?

How much should a private nurse, who has no one dependent on her, save from this sum each year, considering that she has no unusual expenses?

Investing One's Savings.—Not every one who knows how to save knows how to invest the savings wisely, when a certain amount has accumulated. A writer in a magazine* discussing the subject of unwise investments in which the investor emerges minus his hard-earned savings, asks the question, "Who are these dupes?" and answers it as follows:

"The list of names and addresses seized at the fraud offices when an arrest is made shows that they are chiefly school-teachers, widows, clergymen and clerks. The number of women all over the country swindled by mining-stock and patent-right schemers is something appalling. There are no actual statistics on the subject, but the number of gulls and dupes runs up into the millions. In the past five years nearly a hundred million dollars has been sent to New York by these persons, and the money is still coming in at the rate of about fifty thousand dollars a day.

"It is strange that women with their oft-credited 'intuitive minds,' the possession of that wonderful 'sixth sense,' are so easily swindled by glittering circulars and prospectuses."

We would like to believe that nurses are not among the dupes, that they are not easily dazzled by so-called gilt-edge investments, that they are wiser than those who embark in the numerous get-rich-quick schemes. But, unfortunately, we have reason to believe they are not all as wise in the investment of their hard-earned money as they should be. Not long since we learned of over a dozen nurses who had been "bitten" in their attempt to get rich by buying stock in a mine of some kind, supposed to be in Arizona. One nurse had sunk the entire savings of years—over two thousand dollars—in the scheme, and had persuaded others to follow her example. Before long the bubble broke and she was

* The Technical World.

moved to retaliate by instituting a law suit against the stock broker who made the investment for her.

An important ethical question is whether a nurse should ever take the responsibility of inducing other nurses or friends to invest in schemes in which there is a strong element of risk.

When the business is legitimate and at one's door, and apparently a perfectly safe investment, are there reasons why nurses or other wage-earners should hesitate to invest in stock concerns over the management of which they have no control? If so, what are such reasons?

Should a nurse need to use the money which she has invested in a stock concern, how shall she proceed to get it and what difficulties is she likely to encounter?

Ten Rules Concerning Investment.—A magazine* intended especially for the feminine half of the country, gives the following rules regarding investments. Study them carefully. What would you add to them if you were giving a nurse advice regarding how to invest her savings.

1. Six per cent. is a liberal return for the use of money.
2. The higher the interest return, the less safe the investment.
3. Before buying a security find out what you could sell it for if you owned it.
4. Stock extravagantly advertised should never be bought.
5. The personal magnetism of a stock salesman does not add one cent to the value of the stock.
6. Investment, like medicine, is a science practised by experts.
7. Get expert advice concerning investment. You can afford to pay for it, if necessary.

* Woman's Home Companion.

8. The successful banker is the best adviser—when he will advise.

9. Get information about securities from as many sources as possible before buying.

10. Don't invest hurriedly.

Three Bits of Advice.—A very successful business man gives three rules for investors which long experience has taught him should be observed. He says:

"Most failures in life grow out of the unwillingness of a person to profit by the experience of others. My own mistakes would nearly all have been avoided by observing a few simple principles, which I shall endeavor to embody under three short rules.

"RULE I.—*Never loan a needy friend any more money than you can afford to lose.*

"Your friend probably intends in good faith to pay back the money, but the chances are that his schemes will miscarry and he will not be able to repay you.

"RULE II.—*Never invest in a business with which you are not familiar without first having a careful investigation made by disinterested experts of established skill and responsibility.*

"This precaution would save investors from at least nine-tenths of the bad investments that are made.

"RULE III.—*Never take stock or invest in any new enterprise unless you are willing to devote to it your own time and energy.*"

Charities and Free Service.—In every life well lived there will be found running through it, as a golden thread, the expression of the individual's ideals of service in some way. Whether black or white, learned or illiterate, the obligation of service is on us, and the nurse, in common with others, feels or should feel this obligation. To be sure, all nursing is service, but the individual who refuses to render any service for which he is not to receive payment in the coin of the realm misses much of the joy of living and giving. It should be made a matter of principle every year for a nurse to render a certain amount of service for which she never expects to be paid —and we like to believe that most nurses are carrying out the spirit of this principle and rendering free service in a thousand quiet ways and places.

The vexed questions as to whether a nurse should be bound by contract not to work for less than the regulation rate, what treatment should be accorded a nurse who works for less than regular rates, whether a fixed rate or a sliding scale should be adopted—these questions are not to be answered in this volume. Whether the nurse should, when remaining on a long case where the family is undoubtedly having a hard time to meet expenses, lower her rates or give a week's service or two weeks free, is a technical question which cannot be settled by any fixed rule, to which objections cannot be made. But the principle that every nurse in common with every other right-minded individual owes every year some measure of free service to humanity cannot be easily reasoned away.

Nursing in Homes of Moderate Means.—It should, however, be remembered that to the great two-thirds of humanity as we know it in town, city, and country the idea of accepting free service from a nurse is objectionable. The normal life is a life which is lived with the idea of paying, as far as one can, for the commodities and service of others which are received. Dependence on charity is not a wholesome condition, and the spirit of independence and self-respect which is found in the normal life should be cherished by every possible means. Distress may come, periods of adversity may come, when long illness and slack work or unemployment may make the paying of bills a great difficulty or an impossibility, but this does not necessarily mean that a nurse called to nurse in such families should ask them to accept charity. It does mean that she should consider their circumstances and feelings and needs.

A great deal of serious study has been given to the study of how to provide better nursing service for this great two-thirds—the middle-class families living on a moderate income—and the failure of the graduate nurse to understand the spirit of this class of people, to appreciate that their needs can never be met by charity—against which their souls rebel—is responsible in large measure for many perplexing and troublesome conditions relating to nursing, which today are giving serious concern to those who are sincerely interested in nurses, and also in seeing human needs in sickness met in the best possible way.

A graduate nurse marries a man who is earning a salary of $100 a month which must provide rent, food, heat, clothing, care in sickness, etc., for himself, wife and child. What sort of care in sickness is such a woman entitled to in her home, and how should it be provided for her?

The home care in sickness of the great majority of the sick—all classes of sickness—is a question which nurses should carefully study with an open, unprejudiced mind. It is a common mistake to imagine that most of the sick are or can be cared for in hospitals. It is only lately that we have begun to appreciate that, busy and active as are the hospitals, the proportion of people who are ill and cared for in hospitals is small as compared with the whole. In one of the largest cities of the country during the last six months of 1914, even in contagious diseases, more than 79 per cent. of the acute contagious disease patients were cared for at home. The proportion of patients suffering from non-contagious diseases cared for at home is much higher. Investigations carried on in various cities place the proportion of patients who receive hospital care at about 10 per cent. Taking towns and rural districts into such calculations would reduce materially such a percentage. It is an economic mistake to tax the public to erect hospitals for patients who can be adequately cared for at home. The home field offers to the nurse of today her largest opportunity, if only she cultivates a right attitude of mind toward the real needs and shows herself ready to improve her opportunity.

As an illustration of how far we are from providing proper care in sickness even in populous centers where it would seem that medical and nursing care should be easily available, the following figures obtained in an exhaustive survey of a section of a county near New York City are given:

"Of the one hundred and thirteen women who went through childbirth in their homes, only one had the continuous care of a graduate nurse, and only eighteen had any service whatever from visiting nurses. Thirty-five per cent. of the children born came into the world under unfit conditions and surroundings."[1]

What responsibility has the graduate nurse for the existence of such conditions? What should her attitude of mind be in regard to such conditions, and in what ways can she improve them?

What is, or should be, her relation to other workers now in this field?

While it is undoubtedly true that the great two-thirds do not want charity, it is also true that the poor we have always with us, and that occasionally we are called on for

[1] Report made by State Charities Aid Association of New York.

either financial help or free service, or both. The nurse should carefully consider her personal obligations in this matter, and how to wisely distribute such help as she is able to give. Nurses, in common with many other people, are far too prone to appoint a committee to attend to this matter for them and then to consider their duty done.

Suggested Subject for Written Work.—In your opinion can nursing needs in homes of all classes be met by graduate service alone? What suggestions would you make as to the proper way to care for a mother about to give birth to her fifth baby in a small city where the income is $80 a month, the family being several hundreds of miles from any relative.

FOR DISCUSSION OR REVIEW

1. To what extent, if any, is an individual's choice of recreation an index of character? Give illustrations and reasons for your answer.
2. Mention some forms of investment which seem wise for nurses, giving reasons, also the precautions which should be observed regarding them.
3. What are the advantages of life insurance as a form of investment for nurses? What precautions should a nurse use before taking out a life insurance policy?
4. State some different methods of providing for life insurance with some advantages and disadvantages of each method. Give some estimate as to annual payments required in each form.
5. What are the advantages or disadvantages of nurses investing in a business the location of which they have never seen, and which is hundreds of miles from where the investor lives?

6. What are the arguments for or against the fixed rate or the sliding scale for a private nurse?

7. Give some reasons why a nurse should hesitate to offer a self-respecting middle-class family charity?

8. What should be her attitude of mind and what is her responsibility toward this class of people?

9. In a case of minor illness or a chronic ailment, if a practical nurse or untrained worker or attendant assumes the responsibility for the housework and the care of the patient, and the graduate nurse will assume no responsibility beyond the care of the invalid who is only very moderately sick, which worker is the more desirable in that family? Which is worth most to the family? Give reasons for your answer.

10. Can you see any reasons why a physician should choose an untrained woman for such a case?

11. Should a nurse expect to be paid for the time she has spent in training, or for the service she actually renders in a home?

12. Mention some reasons why the home field offers to the nurse of today a large opportunity for service.

13. Suggest some methods by which improvement in present-day conditions might be accomplished.

14. What has the attitude of mind of the individual nurse to do with this great problem?

CHAPTER XXIII

Ethical Problems in Private Nursing

It is probable that in no branch of nursing do more perplexing ethical problems arise than in private nursing. In a hospital, and in visiting nursing, there are general rules of guidance that help a nurse to steer clear of many pitfalls, and there is usually some experienced worker to appeal to for advice. In a hospital, also, the nurse is surrounded with all sorts of conveniences for her work. In private nursing the conditions vary with each individual case, and the nurse must frequently decide questions of large importance without a chance to talk the matter over with anybody.

In the hospital it is essential that a nurse be systematic in her work, that she make a careful division of her time between several patients, that she carefully observe orders and regulations and develop a certain amount of speed in getting through with duties according to a prescribed method.

In the field of private nursing a nurse must be able to get along with few orders, must regulate her own habits and methods according to the situation in which she finds herself, must know how to get along with the patient and his friends without antagonizing them, and must show a willingness to do whatever she finds necessary that will add to the comfort or recovery of the patient.

It is well for a nurse to remember that the financial success of a private nurse depends greatly on whether or not she so conducts herself in the homes of her patients that they will recommend her to her friends. No nurses are so dependent on this matter of recommendations as private nurses. A satisfied patient and family is a nurse's best advertisement. Her technical skill counts for much less in the estimation of many families than the thousand and one little things which she may do every day that will keep things running smoothly, and the patient as happy and contented as can be under the circumstances. A patient is not usually either greatly interested in or deeply appreciative of a nurse's knowledge of embryology or bacteriology, but he is intensely interested in how his egg is cooked, how his beefsteak is served, whether his tea or coffee is to his liking, whether his tray comes with salt, pepper, butter or some other item missing, thus causing him exasperating delays. He may ply a nurse with questions about the hospital, the doctors, or about former patients, and then after she has satisfied him that she has no objection to freely discussing these subjects, he will tell his friends that she is a great gossip, and that a nurse who will talk to him about other patients and their affairs will carry tales about his affairs to others and they had better not employ her.

The variety of ethical problems that arise in private homes is exhaustless, but most of them will fit into one of the following classes:

Problems for which the nurse herself is responsible.

Problems directly connected with the patient.

Problems relating to the family and domestic situation.

Problems relating chiefly to the doctor.

The remainder may be classed under the head of "miscellaneous."

Responses to Calls.—The most frequent complaints about private nurses are heard in regard to the questions of responses to calls, to her unwillingness to wait on herself or to do anything not directly connected with the care of the patient, and to her extravagance. These are types of problems for which the nurse herself is responsible. Very frequently she takes her cue in these matters from some other nurse whose example should be avoided rather than followed, instead of seriously asking herself "What is my duty in this case? If the Golden Rule were followed, what course would it lead me to pursue?"

A doctor who has had a wide experience with private nurses states emphatically his opinion of the nurse's professional obligations in regard to responses to calls in this manner: "A nurse who has reported that she is on call or who is not actually on duty is as much bound, ethically and professionally, to respond to a doctor's call for a nurse as is a doctor to respond to a call for his professional service."

If this doctor's view of the nurse's professional obligations were subscribed to and practised by nurses in general, what desirable or undesirable results would be likely to follow?

To what extent and at what time in her career is it desirable for a nurse to specialize?

What limitations should she make regarding what cases she will or will not take and what times she will and will not work?

Having made limitations and announced them, is a nurse under obligation to observe them?

When a nurse announces herself as "on call" for "general nursing" what does she mean? Does she mean that she is ready to respond to any call that comes? If not, what does she mean by "general nursing?"

What does it mean to be "on call," and what limitations does a nurse place on her own plans and movements when she has announced that she is "on call?"

Should a nurse on private duty be either absolutely "on call" or absolutely not "on call?"

Would the adherence to a rule requiring a nurse to be either absolutely "on call" or absolutely not "on call" settle some of the perplexing questions in nursing that arise? We think it would. To be "on call" only for an easy or so-called "good case" or for a favorite doctor is perhaps the chief thing which physicians condemn, and rightly condemn, in nurses. A rule to do general nursing and to be "on call" or not "on call" absolutely, and a determination to give prompt response to any call at any time or place when one is "on call," is one of the best rules that a young nurse can make, due regard being made to the matter of just remuneration.

A rule to be "on call" or not "on call" absolutely gives a nurse large command over her time, and makes it possible for her to secure the rest periods that she needs.

The charge of "picking cases," which is so detrimental to the whole nursing body, would never have been made had trained nurses adhered to the principle of absolutely being "on call" and ready to respond, or absolutely not "on call." This evil can be remedied only as the individual nurse resolves to remedy it in herself, and to use her influence to help other nurses to realize their professional obligations in this matter.

The absolutely unethical conditions which prevail in many places may be illustrated by the following: A doctor requires a nurse for a boy fourteen years old. The boy lives with his parents in a comfortable home five miles beyond the city limits, easily reached by trolley car. The first nurse called "didn't care to go out of the city." The second called had made an engagement to go to the theatre. Would tomorrow do? The third nurse "didn't care to nurse children." The fourth had just had a short case and didn't wish to take another. The fifth would go, but her clean linen had not come from the laundry and she hadn't a thing to wear. The sixth had a headache, but if she felt better might go tomorrow.

It is nothing unusual to call fifteen nurses for some serious case of this kind before getting one who is ready to respond, while all have reported themselves as "on call." It is hardly to be wondered at that doctors tire of this attitude and refuse to call such nurses for any case. Nor is it to be wondered at that such nurses are idle a good part of the time, and thoroughly discontented with conditions.

Practically the same conditions are met with by the registrars who manage registries for nurses. Nurses report that they are "on call," yet when a call comes they have a dozen questions to ask about it, then finally decide they do not care to take it.

Specializing is entirely proper and the only ethical way of limiting responses to calls. If a nurse wishes to register for "surgical cases only" or for other cases only, that is her privilege. There is nothing unprofessional about it, but when she begins to ennumerate the kinds of cases she *will not go to,* she leaves the impression that she regards no obligations to the profession or to the sick, that she is unwilling to sacrifice her personal convenience under any circumstances, that she is going to do just as little as she can possibly manage, and that she is influenced wholly by selfish or personal motives. Consistent adherence to the professional limitations which she has made in regard to her calls is the chief ethical requirement in such cases.

The dilatory nurse is always a trial to doctors, to those who are in charge of her calls and to those who employ her. She is never quite ready to at once respond to a call, or she has developed a habit of "dilly-dallying" over her preparations, or she deliberately refuses to go at once to a case by the shortest route and in the shortest possible time. In any case the results are exasperating and often serious. A doctor is called to a case of uterine hemorrhage. He uses emergency measures, telephones for a nurse who says she will be there at the earliest possible moment. He expects her in less than an hour. He is afraid to leave the patient till she comes. One hour, two and sometimes three hours pass before the nurse appears with an assortment of excuses and explanations ready to present. The doctor's duties and appointments are interfered with, and those of many other people who had appointments with him. What should be a doctor's attitude toward this type of nurse?

The most reprehensible fact about the dilatory nurse is that she often deliberately delays going to a case after she has agreed to go. A nurse stated her policies to the author in this manner: "I am never in any hurry about getting to a new case. I find that people respect you more if you don't act as if you were too glad to get the call, or as if you were sitting waiting for it." The condition or needs of the patient seemed to be an entirely secondary consideration with this nurse. It was herself, and how she was to be received, that was uppermost in her thought and plans. What important ethical qualities for a nurse were lacking in the case just cited?

Economy and Nursing.—The charge of extravagance is so frequently heard about nurses that measures to guard against it should be seriously considered by every nurse. It is one of the chief reasons why many families who could afford to pay a graduate nurse prefer an untrained or practical nurse, because the latter is usually more careful regarding general expenses.

True economy is not stinginess. "It is a far-seeing, clear-sighted grasp of all the possibilities of a situation, and a habit of mind which secures the maximum advantage from every fraction of outlay, whether in energy or cash, which are frequently interchangeable terms. True economy conduces to comfort, while false economy is the essence of discomfort."

Quite often the really good work that a nurse does on a case is forgotten because it was expected and taken for granted, while some bit of carelessness or extravagance is remembered and talked about because it was unworthy of a trained woman. A nurse wrapped a baby in an expensive blanket, sat too near a grate fire with it, and burned a fairly large hole in the blanket. So long as that patched blanket remains, the story of that nurse's carelessness will be told.

Quite often a nurse fails to provide herself with a good practical working outfit which every nurse should have, and calls on every family to which she goes to purchase things which she expects to need frequently and should carry with her.

Too lavish use of linen is a common complaint, and in many cases the laundry bills seem to be out of all proportion to real needs. One difficulty with the whole matter of economy is that, while in training, nurses are constantly using expensive articles for which they do not pay, and they leave the training school ignorant of what waste means, or of how the cost of common articles mounts up when combined with the other added expenses of sickness. Many nurses are experts at improvising. Bed-rests, cradles, supports, heating appliances, croup kettles and tents, foot baths, drinking cups, urinals, measuring glasses, etc., are all produced without cost. Every nurse should take pride in being able to improvise such things. She may not need to do it in all cases, but she should know how to meet needs as they arise.

The marring of costly furniture—dresser tops or tables—by setting hot water pitchers on them or by spilling water or chemicals on them, and not quickly wiping it off, or by wet-dusting, is another danger point which nurses do well to guard against.

A nurse writer in one of the nursing magazines cites this incident which illustrates admirably the impression made in some homes by nurses who offend by their carelessness.

"A friend recently told me with horror in her eyes that she had just had a trained nurse who had actually spilled olive oil on her bath-room rug and the spots would not come out. 'Why,' said she, 'I, who have never been in a hospital, used it myself for weeks without spilling a drop!' Alas for that nurse! Of what use has her training been to her if she occasionally spills olive oil? As long as the bath-room rug exists in that home the name of nurse will not mean the sweet-faced, ministering angel, the tower of strength, the kindly presence. No, it suggests but one thing—unremovable, unfadable, unpardonable spots!"

Very often at first sight it looks as though there is no way to avoid considerable expense if the sick one is to be made comfortable, yet it can often be done. A nurse called to nurse a young man in the country, ill with typhoid fever, was distressed to find the sick-room and house swarming with flies. There were no screens on the house and she explained the danger from the flies, and the necessity of screens. It was harvest time and nobody on the farm had time to make screens. The people were deeply in debt and said they simply could not afford the cost of screening the house. Several yards of mosquito netting had been bought, part of which had been used to throw over the patient. The nurse pondered over the matter, and next morning undertook the screening herself. She tacked pieces of the netting over the lower half of the windows in the sick-room, and with the remainder she made a curtain for the door of the room, tacking it at the top and on one side. She then instituted a "swat-the-fly" campaign in the room, and in a few hours had the room clear of flies without a cent of extra expense. Thousands of nurses have shown similar and very commendable ingenuity in keeping expense down, yet doing the needed things.

Quite frequently a nurse on going to a home will find that the family themselves have exhibited little sense in regard to sickness, and that their devotion is expressed in very unwise ways. A young woman will often supply an expensive layette for the coming baby, and fail to supply herself with sufficient nightdresses; or some member of the family will invest in an expensive coat or ring for the child when there is real need of sheets for the mother's bed. These are trying occasions to meet, but at least the nurse should be able while there to give such a family better notions of true economy.

In many families a spirit of recklessness regarding expenditures develops owing to misguided devotion. Useless and unnecessary expense is incurred, the effect of which will be felt long after the illness has passed. Too often the whole blame for this reckless extravagance is laid on the nurse, and the family, handicapped by pressing bills, resolves never to have a trained nurse in the house again. By tactful management, the nurse can often persuade a family that some proposed expense is needless.

A short time ago the writer was told of a nurse who donned a clean white dress every day, sent the dresses to the laundry, and added her laundry bill in every case to her regular charges. Such nurses do more to prejudice the public against trained nurses than a score of sensible conscientious nurses can undo. What do they expect to gain by such conduct? Is there any way to check the growth of such practices?

Suggested Subject for Written Work.—A private nurse made the statement that a graduate nurse is no more under obligation to accept a call to a case unless it happens to suit her than is a carpenter to accept an opportunity which is offered him to build a house unless the conditions were satisfactory to him. Contrast this mental attitude of the nurse with Florence Nightingale's ideals of service. Tell why you do or do not agree with this nurse's position in the question under consideration. What is the meaning of the phrase "professional obligations?" Is this nurse practising a profession or a trade?

FOR DISCUSSION OR REVIEW

Estimate the cost to a family, living on an income of $125 a month, of an illness from typhoid fever lasting six weeks. The woman assists and relieves the nurse; the man is the patient. A maid is secured at $5 a week. Include in your estimate doctor's calls, drugs of all kinds, extra laundry, extra food supplies for the sick, for the maid and the nurse, loss of wages, trained nurse's salary, board of nurse and servant, and such incidental expenses as you think are necessary in a middle-class home.

A nurse carried a fruit knife, which a patient had presented to her, with her when she went to nurse in a private home. Accidentally she threw the fruit knife with some orange peelings into the grate, and before she discovered it the knife was ruined. The patient knew nothing of the occurrence till a bill for $2.50 was presented to him by the nurse for the knife which through her own carelessness she had destroyed. In what moral qualities was this nurse lacking?

Under what circumstances is a nurse who has applied to doctors and through a registry for general nursing justified in refusing to nurse patients ill with acute contagious diseases?

Is a nurse justified in accepting engagements for obstetrical cases with the provision that she has no other case when the call comes?

A nurse makes an engagement for an obstetrical case for probably a certain week. The obstetrical case calls her three weeks before the expected time. She is employed on a pneumonia case. Should she leave to keep her engagement with the obstetrical patient?

A nurse in a western state was called to a case of typhoid fever on a farm in an isolated section. The family was hardworking, ignorant, and lacking in the first principles of cleanliness. The bed was wooden and infested with bed-bugs which bothered both nurse and patient, who slept on another wooden bed in the same room. The nurse told the family she would have to have a new bed for herself and one for the patient that was free from bugs. They paid no attention to her request, so she wrote to a firm in the city ordering an iron bed and mattress for the patient, a cot and mattress for herself, rubber sheeting, several basins, ice-caps, etc., having the bill sent to the family. When she presented her bill the family paid part of it, but deducted the amount of the bill for the articles which she had ordered without their knowledge or consent. She sued for the remainder of her bill. The newspaper notoriety in the case affected her and other nurses in the region adversely. Was her course of action in regard to the case commendable or otherwise? What different methods should she have pursued?

If called to nurse an obstetrical patient in a home with an income of $100 a month, what articles would you ask the prospective mother to provide for the sickness? Itemize the cost of the different articles and estimate the total cost of the sickness.

Outline what you would consider a nurse's duties in such a home where there is a child two and a half years of age.

CHAPTER XXIV

Ethical Problems in Private Nursing

(Continued)

Nurses probably more than any other class of workers see the inside of people's lives and the seamy as well as the happy side of domestic situations. The nurse's greatest difficulty arises as a rule in determining the exact extent of her duty in the home she has entered. Shall she set for herself a certain routine of duties which she deems to be all that the patient or family have a right to demand, or shall she give consideration to the problems of each individual household and try to do her best for each situation?

The question of dignity frequently arises in the mind of a nurse. She is perhaps afraid if she does this, that, or the other thing, she will be less respected, or she has been told that she will be imposed on, and consequently serves notice on the family in a dozen indirect ways that "they need not think they can impose on me." Her perplexity increases perhaps as she relates her experience in one home to some older nurse friend and the friend perhaps criticizes her for doing some small thing, which took but little time or effort, but relieved the patient's mind, a thing which was simply an ordinary kindness. The inexperienced nurse who really wants to follow the Golden Rule and who really wants to fulfil her pledge which stated "That into whatsoever house you shall enter, it shall be for the good of the sick to the utmost of your power," who interprets this pledge literally, really means to keep it, is often seriously disturbed because of the criticisms of older nurses, and wonders whether she has done something "unprofessional."

A young graduate on her first obstetrical case was asked by the young mother if she would wash out the baby's fine woolen shirts in the bathroom, and stretch them carefully while drying. The mother did not want to send them to the laundry. The maid-of-all-work was a foreigner, who did not understand English very well, and the mother was afraid to trust her with the little shirts, which she expected to take care of herself when she was out of bed. The young nurse was not sure whether this duty came in her province or not, but she finally decided to do it, and then try to find out what the custom of other nurses was in regard to such matters. The incident assumed an importance in her mind out of all proportion to the matter involved, which was a simple act of kindness. Two nurses whom she consulted said she should not have done it, that she was "lowering the standards of the profession," a third one thought she did right, said she would have done the same thing. To settle the disputed question, the young nurse finally wrote to the office of a nursing magazine for an opinion as to whether she did right or wrong to wash out those little shirts. The whole question was so unimportant as to seem unworthy of any earnest sincere group of women, who desired to be treated as professional people.

The nurse who really desires to keep her promise to labor "for the good of the sick to the utmost of her power" will wisely settle such questions, by adopting a resolution the spirit of which is "I will do such necessary duties as present themselves, whole-heartedly and gladly. I will not neglect the opportunity to perform acts of everyday kindness that come to me." Considering incidental duties which are not strictly nursing, as "acts of kindness, thrown in for good measure" will help a nurse in the long run, more than she can possibly realize. It is still true that "with what measure ye mete, it shall be measured to you again."

Another rule of thought which expresses the spirit which a nurse should carry into her work is this: "There is nothing which needs to be done for the comfort of any patient which it is beneath my dignity to do."

When Florence Nightingale began her work, it was necessary to educate the public to a higher conception of nursing than the world had ever known. It was necessary to draw a more or less distinct line between the duties of a nurse and the duties of a domestic servant. Then, female labor was cheaply and easily secured. Most middle-class families who did not employ servants had some "unattached" relative who could help in times of sickness in the home. But a half century has wrought marked social changes. Opportunities for women to become wage-earners have greatly multiplied, and household helpers in the home are less readily secured. Labor-saving ideas have been applied to the home. Flat-dwellings and apartment houses have simplified household duties, so that domestic servants are not needed or employed in the great majority of homes. The social status of the nurse has been established. All these changes should have wrought corresponding changes in the nurse's outlook on her duties, but there are thousands of nurses who refuse to move or change with the times, who have very false notions of dignity, and very exaggerated ideas of the deference which should be shown to their position. The list of things which they will not do in homes often far exceeds the list of duties which they will do. One physician in speaking of a certain nurse stated that "she was too classical to see anything to do;" so the family dispensed quickly with her services. It is such nurses who complain that the field of nursing is overcrowded. Without doubt, parts of the field are overcrowded by this type of nurse, but for the nurse with a vision, the nurse who is willing, kind, industrious, and tactful, as well as skilled in technic, the field is ever broadening.

Too much dignity leads to poor nursing very often, which the following incident will illustrate:

A young graduate was engaged to nurse an obstetrical patient on the fifth floor of an apartment hotel. The nurse was to have her meals in the common dining room in the basement of the hotel, and the patient's meals were to be served from the hotel kitchen. The arrangement seemed admirable. The working out was abominable. The nurse assumed no responsibility about the patient's tray, and at nearly every meal something was missing that caused exasperating delays. The nurse rang for the elevator man to carry messages to the kitchen, waited for him to come, told him perhaps that tea had been sent when it should have been coffee, or that the salt or butter was missing. The elevator man carried the message to the kitchen workers. They were busy about other things, and did not always respond at once. Meantime the food on the patient's tray was cooling and the result was that the meals were most unsatisfactory affairs, when a little less dignity, and a little more effort on the part of the nurse, would have resulted in satisfactory meals and a contented instead of disgruntled patient.

The same nurse monopolized the bath room each morning for nearly an hour, taking a morning bath, and dressing her hair elaborately and leisurely, while the husband fumed about it to his wife, because he couldn't get into the bath room to shave before going to his work. After the second morning that this happened, he was going to dismiss the nurse, and only the pleadings of his wife to avoid "a fuss" prevented his doing so.

The same nurse was most unaccommodating so far as the maids were concerned. She was always busy bathing the baby or attending to the patient when the maid came to clean the room, and the result was that the husband complained at the office that their rooms were neglected. The family, after she was gone, announced to their doctor and friends that never again would they employ a nurse trained in Blank training school.

Comment on this nurse's management of the situation and show where her real failures were. What desirable qualities did she lack? Outline what you would consider a good method of managing such a situation.

The arrangements about meals are the cause of many disagreements that arise between nurse and family, which difficulties, practically always, react to the disadvantage of the nurse. A nurse is entirely justified in refusing to go to the kitchen for meals with the servants, but is she always justified in demanding that she be treated as a guest in the home? Many nurses seem to feel that the family that is employing them owes them exactly the same attention and deference that would be shown to a guest. A nurse in advising a young private nurse as to what to do and what to refuse to do in a home remarked to her, that she always took an "evening gown" with her to every case, and always "dressed for dinner." Naturally such a nurse is discontented when a family occasionally desires to have a dinner without her, while she is in the home. This false idea of a nurse's real position and mission in a home is the cause of the loss of many hundreds of dollars a year to nurses. Two illustrations are typical of the way in which such difficulties react adversely on the nurse herself.

A nurse was called to nurse a patient in a wealthy home. The illness was of a chronic nature, with occasional periods in which the patient suffered considerably, and needed some special care for weeks at a time. As the illness progressed, the services of a nurse were needed practically all the time, though the duties were very light. The young people of the family wished to entertain friends at meals frequently, and asked the mother to arrange for the nurse to take her meals before or after the regular meals in the dining room. The nurse rebelled against this arrangement. The family waited till the end of her week, dispensed with her services, and called an untrained or practical nurse to the case. The nurse lost a case that would have lasted for months, where the family were able and willing to keep her, and a case in which her work was about as light as it could possibly be. What did she gain? Was her position in the matter right or wrong?

In another case, the patient, an elderly gentleman, had had a slight stroke of paralysis. The family were wealthy, and quite nervous about further attacks, and employed two nurses, so that the patient would always have some one within call, night and day. He was recovering, and able to sit up in a chair most of the day, when the family had several visitors arrive at their summer home, where the patient was. The family felt they would prefer not to have the nurses at the table, and offered to serve their meals on trays on a small table in a room adjoining the patient's room, or else have the nurses come to a second table in the family dining room. The nurses objected to either arrangement. They felt they should come to the family table with the guests.

The result was that the family telephoned to a near-by city for a male nurse who would do all that needed to be done for the patient night or day, and take his meals at a second table, and the two nurses were told that their services would be no longer required.

What general principles should guide a nurse in settling the question of arrangements for meals? What are her rights in this matter?

Domestic problems usually increase for the nurse, very decidedly when the woman who is head of the home becomes the patient. When the woman is in general charge, affairs are apt to move along more evenly. A difficulty that sometimes arises is due to jealousy when the husband is the patient. Quite frequently there is absolutely no reason for such jealousy. At other times the nurse's methods and manner are such as to arouse prejudice against her. She perhaps objects to the wife being in the room at certain times, or her manner and tones are a shade too familiar. A nurse was employed to nurse a young husband who had typhoid fever. The young couple were very devoted to each other, and at intervals during the day the wife would sit by the bedside holding the patient's hand, petting him in various ways and calling him by endearing terms. The nurse foolishly allowed herself to fall into the habit of using some of the same endearing terms as the wife did. She called the man by his Christian name before she had been in the house a half day. When she came to take temperature and pulse after the wife had been holding his hand, she would remark "Now it is my turn to hold your hand." The sick man himself was disgusted with her familiar way of talking, his wife became jealous, and at the end of the first week the nurse was sent away and another nurse called.

Tone and Manner.—It is hard to make some nurses realize that their relation to men patients has no counterpart in ordinary life. There must be new rules of conduct, and no nurse can too soon learn the importance that tone and manner assume in such relations. Thoughtless acts which may have a perfectly innocent intention back of them are apt to be misconstrued. Is it ever proper for a nurse to call an adult male patient in his home by his Christian name? What rules should a nurse observe in this respect?

Difficulties with servants can usually be avoided if a nurse is careful to make requests and avoid commands, and if she takes pains to speak the kind words which do so much to keep the domestic machinery running smoothly. If the nurse is careful not to impose on the servant, or make unnecessary demands on her, is kind, obliging, and tactful, friction will rarely occur.

Temperamental difficulties in families frequently occur which tax the nurse's ingenuity to the utmost. For example: The patient is a young man and an only child. His mother is a widow. His disease is empyema and the nurse is on the case for more than two months. His mother is nervous and apprehensive about the patient and wants to be with him as much as possible. Her presence is distinctly depressing to the patient and tends to make him nervous and to worry over his condition. He admits this to the nurse, but insists that his mother must not know that her presence affects him as it does. How can the nurse manage this situation so that the young man has the best possible chance for a comfortable and speedy recovery, and the mother is not offended or made suspicious that the nurse is trying to keep her out of the sick-room?

Ethical difficulties in which doctors are concerned are of frequent occurrence, and a nurse's chance for future work can often be affected disastrously, if a doctor has reason to suspect her disloyalty or if she appears to be overstepping what he considers to be her professional province. It is a rather one-sided loyalty frequently that the physician demands. He often sees no reason why he should be loyal to the nurse, while he is quick to condemn her for apparent disloyalty to him.

Not infrequently, a nurse is torn between her desire to be loyal to the patient's interests, and not disloyal to the doctor, who has it in his power to turn calls in her direction and to influence other doctors to do the same, or the reverse. Doctors are loath to admit that loyalty to the patient's welfare is ever incompatible with the loyalty which a nurse has been taught she must render to a physician. The following quotation from an eminent New York physician probably states what most physicians believe: "Loyalty to the physician and faithfulness to the patient do not form a twofold proposition, but a single one, for supposing that the nurse detected the physician in an erroneous course of treatment, she should so notify him at once." Unfortunately, theory and practice are not always in accord, and the difficulty is by no means so easily disposed of as the distinguished physician imagines. It is, however, well that nurses should understand how physicians look at the matter, and proceed cautiously in doubtful situations.

Does loyalty to the physician and faithfulness to the patient always mean one and the same thing?

A nurse is called to care for a patient who appears to be suffering from some abdominal trouble. The patient is of a nervous type and has been operated on for abdominal trouble less than two years previously. The doctor suggests another operation. The patient protests against it and the doctor demands that a consultant be called.

He is given permission to choose his own consultant and they exactly agree as to diagnosis and treatment. The husband of the patient is far from satisfied that an operation is needed. The nurse is not supposed to diagnose, but she can hardly help forming an opinion as to whether the operation is as urgently needed as the doctor suggests. The patient and husband both look to her for some suggestion. What should she do?

A nurse is called to nurse a case of septicemia following abortion. The patient, a young married woman, is very ill, and confesses to the nurse that she wished she had never had the abortion performed. It is evident that the doctor in charge of the case is the one who secured the abortion, though the patient does not plainly say so. The doctor appears to be attentive to the case, but thoroughly incompetent. The nurse feels that under different management the patient might have a chance to recover. What is her duty in the matter?

A patient had been ill for several months, and had suffered many things of many physicians. The diagnosis differed with each physician. Finally she died. The husband had paid large bills for physician's services and was determined to have a post-mortem examination made, to find out the real cause of death. He privately told the nurse that he had no faith in the physician in charge of the case at death, and tolerated him only because his wife liked him. The husband has a suspicion that the physician who did the post-mortem examination might refuse to reveal the true findings and might make the post-mortem findings agree with his diagnosis made during the illness. The husband asks the nurse to be present at the post-mortem and report the truth to him. What should she do?

A nurse in charge of a patient with a chronic illness is

instructed to keep the physician informed as to the patient's condition. The patient grows dissatisfied with the physician; the nurse feeling that the change from day to day is very slight, does not communicate with the physician nor report the patient's growing dissatisfaction with the treatment. Another physician is called. Wherein was the nurse at fault?

A nurse is engaged to travel with a patient. The doctor tells the nurse that the patient requires no treatment but just ordinary care. At the last moment before starting the nurse learns that the doctor has deceived her, that the patient has been having and is expected to have long and somewhat difficult treatments every day which are hard to manage in hotels and while traveling. What should she do?

A family engages a nurse for an obstetrical case, telling her the name of the physician who will be in charge of the case. Before the birth the family change physicians owing to some business reasons, and the physician who will have charge of the case is one whom the nurse distrusts professionally, and dislikes personally. Should she go on with the case? If not, what reason should she give the family for refusing?

A nurse is called to a hotel to care for an elderly gentleman who has been taken ill while traveling. He is 1500 miles from his family. He does not improve. The doctor makes light of his illness, tells the patient he is going to get well, and when asked by the patient if there is any danger, that if there is he would like to make his will, is told there is absolutely no danger. The family expect the nurse to keep them informed of the patient's condition. The doctor, apparently for no reason, insists that she shall tell the family that the patient is improving daily. The nurse knows he is failing steadily.

She fears death cannot be very far off. What is her duty in the case?

A patient is told by a friend that some one has been helped of a disease similar to his, by a certain medicine. He asks the doctor if he can be given that medicine. The doctor agrees, because the patient seems to greatly desire it. He prepares a placebo and tells the nurse she is to tell the patient that this is the medicine he asked for. The nurse objects. The doctor tells her that it is a case where a lie is justifiable and she must tell the patient that this is the medicine his friend recommended. What should the nurse do?

A nurse who had been accustomed to accompanying doctors when they visited patients in their rooms in a hospital, felt she must carry the same rule of procedure into private homes. A lady patient complained that the nurse watched her like a cat and never let her have a word in private with any one, until she finally had to ask her to leave the room when she wished to have a private conversation with the doctor who was an old family friend. Should a nurse always remain in a room in a private home while a doctor is making his visit? What general rules of procedure should she observe in such cases, with the doctor, with the family?

A nurse is employed on a case when a doctor, who frequently calls for her services, asks her to take a case for him; he tells her they will wait a few days for her if necessary. The family in which she is nursing think she can be spared at the end of the week, and she arranges on that basis. Meantime the patient develops a rather serious complication, needs her, and the doctor in charge is unwilling to let her go to the other case as agreed. Should the nurse stay?

A patient under treatment of one doctor calls another

physician without suggesting to the first doctor his desire to change. The patient claims that he has as much right to go to whom he chooses and when he chooses for medical treatment, as he has to go to a different grocer. He had told the first doctor that when he wanted him to call again he would let him know, and he considers that is sufficient. What is the nurse's duty in the case?

How would you improvise substitutes for the following hospital appliances: bed-rest; bed-pan; douche-pan; rubber air cushion; rubber sheeting; ice-cap; hot-water bottle for application of heat to abdomen; croup kettle; measuring glass for urine; fountain syringe; dressing basin; screen. Estimate the cost of these hospital appliances, if bought through a neighborhood drug store, or retail establishment in your own vicinity.

A nurse is called to nurse a child critically ill with pneumonia. The family wish her to apply onion poultices to the feet, and to rub a certain ointment on the chest. The treatments will probably not do any harm. What should the nurse do about it?

Is it possible for a nurse to literally obey the rule, never to diagnose and never to prescribe? If a child is taken suddenly ill in the night with a suspicious-sounding cough, and labored breathing, what might she suspect, and what should she do? What working rules may a nurse adopt to guide her in such situations?

A nurse who had been caring for a seriously ill patient in his home was dismissed, and another nurse substituted. The first nurse took away with her the clinical records which she had kept and refused to return them, until threatened with a law suit. She claimed that the records belonged to her. The doctor claimed that they belonged to the patient—that the keeping of clinical records was a part of the professional service, which the nurse had been paid to render. Rather than allow the question of ownership to go to the courts, the nurse gave up the records. Which party was right in this matter?

CHAPTER XXV

Miscellaneous Problems in Ethics

Among the ethical problems which arise before graduation, disciplinary problems loom up large. However carefully nurses are taught, and however fine and noble are the human examples placed before nurses, it is impossible, sometimes, to have important rules observed unless penalties are attached. Various forms of self-government in schools of nursing have been tried and the plan has much to commend it. One principal in a Canadian school has instituted a Council of Honor, or Court of Honor, on which representatives of the different classes in training have a place. A variety of ethical problems are referred to the pupils for consideration and a feeling of responsibility for maintaining the honor of the school is developed by the consideration of real problems in ethics on which their judgment is asked.

1. A principal who had great difficulty in regard to punctuality at breakfast, finding that admonitions had little effect, instituted a roll call, and a rule that failure to report in the dining room promptly at the appointed hour, twice, would deprive the nurse of her afternoon off duty for the week following the second time the nurse was late, or tried to go on duty without breakfast.

Was this method of discipline wise or unwise? Can you suggest other methods of discipline more suitable for dealing with this condition?

2. A doctor became very angry with a senior pupil nurse, because she answered a patient's questions as to

what, had been done in a certain abdominal operation. He demanded that the pupil nurse be dismissed from the school within twenty-four hours or he would set in motion machinery to have the superintendent, who was also the principal of the school, removed. The superintendent's position in the hospital (a fifty-bed institution) was exceedingly difficult, owing to one-man control on the board, and to the fact that the one man in actual control invited petty gossip and complaints about the institution to come to his office, and every doctor knew this. The nurse in question was within four months of graduation. The superintendent decided to suspend the nurse till the storm which she had caused had subsided, let her return to finish her term, and to place her on night duty, in the children's ward, and in other places where she would not encounter the doctor who demanded her dismissal. Discuss this method of dealing with this situation, and of dealing with similar situations, in which nurses create trouble with the tongue. Suggest ways of impressing nurses with the necessity of diligent control of the little unruly member.

3. A young principal of a training school, in her first position, believed that a training school should be "ruled by love" and was opposed to written or printed rules, regulations or by-laws of any kind for the guidance of head nurses and pupil nurses. Is there anything incompatible between "ruling by love" and having definite rules of guidance? Mention some difficulties which pupils might experience who were in their probation period in a large school with no rules or regulations about anything, outside the orders which related to patients?

4. A pupil nurse who was assisting in an out-patient department of a large hospital, by neglecting to carefully

read the label on a bottle, accidentally caused a patient to be burned with carbolic acid. The disciplinary method used in her case was as follows: The nurse was suspended for two weeks from duty, was obliged to remain in the city and go every day to apply a dressing to the wound which she had caused. Discuss this method of discipline with regard to its probable effect on the nurse, the school, the patient, and the hospital.

5. The question of rank or seniority in a certain small school had for many years been decided by the day or hour at which pupils arrived. A serious situation developed because for some misdemeanor a nurse, who had been the senior in rank in her class, was deprived of her rank and placed at the foot, and a nurse whom she disliked was promoted to first place. These two nurses who were fiercely jealous of each other, were in charge of a seriously ill patient. They refused to cooperate on the case or even to speak to each other. The patient died. The principal impressed with the seriousness of the situation which developed, decided in future to determine seniority or rank in a class by the record made in theoretical and practical work during probation, and to let the record the nurse made each year in observance of rules, care of room, general deportment, and theoretical and practical work, fix her rank in the class and school. Which method of determining rank seems best, and why?

6. A pupil nurse in her senior year in a hospital was placed on operating-room duty. She hated operating-room work, she said, and could see no reason why she should ever have to do it. In what way would her attitude toward the operating-room work be likely to affect the quality of her work? What should the principal do in such a case? It is necessary or desirable for every

nurse to spend a fixed term of training in the operating room? Give reasons for or against.

7. A nurse who had just completed a post-graduate course was employed to take the place of a supervisor of nurses who was given a two months' vacation. The school was connected with a special hospital of over 100 beds, and having affiliation for medical nursing experience with a large hospital. The nurse, who was supplying for the supervisor, had a prejudice against all training schools connected with special hospitals, and told the pupil nurses how strongly she felt on the subject. She established confidential relations with several of the pupils, and in confidence told them they were wasting their time in such a school and she would advise them to leave and seek admission into a certain hospital where she claimed to have influence with the superintendent. She even went so far, while she was employed by the special hospital, as to write out recommendations for the three nurses in whom she was particularly interested, for them to send with their applications, promising to write recommendations for other pupil nurses if these three applications were accepted. Comment on this incident stating why you approve or disapprove of this head nurse's conduct.

8. Should a pupil nurse who is habitually untidy about her room and lax in regard to neatness in her general work be allowed to graduate? How can such habits be corrected? How can a principal be sure that, even if temporary improvement is made, such a nurse will not bring discredit on the school by her untidiness in private homes?

9. A graduate nurse is engaged by a doctor for special duty with an obstetrical patient in a hospital. She seems devoted to the mother and baby and the general

nursing care is good, but in the two weeks she was on duty in the hospital, the room was never tidy. The baby's things were scattered on radiators, chairs, window sills, dresser and every other available spot on which things could conveniently be dropped. Before leaving, this nurse asks the principal to give her other calls for special duty? What should the principal do? How will the example of this graduate affect the pupils in training?

10. A nurse who has an unusual memory is able to pass written examinations taking a full 100 per cent. in many, and a high grade in all. Her practical work is very inferior. She seems to lack judgment and tact and is not always truthful. What should the principal do in regard to this case? What points should be considered? Which is more important, the theoretical knowledge a nurse possesses, or the way she does her work? Give reasons for your answer.

11. A principal of a large training school, writing on ideals for nurses, expresses herself as follows: "It does not seem to me that the probationer who tucks her napkin in her collar will make the kind of nurse we want to send out into the world, nor does it seem to me that it is my function to instruct her in the matter." Is the fact that a probationer "tucks her napkin in her collar" a sufficient reason for rejecting her, if she is acceptable otherwise? If she is accepted as a nurse, whose business is it to call attention to such breaches of etiquette?

12. A nurse through carelessness caused a patient to be burned with a hot-water bottle. In order to impress her with the seriousness of her failure the principal took away her cap for a month. She rebelled against this treatment and left the school. A little later she meekly applied to be reinstated. What should the principal do?

ETHICS AND VISITING NURSING

13. A visiting nurse making a call at a home is asked by the keeper of a rooming house next door to see a young man who has a room there and who is ill. The landlady of the rooming house has called a neighborhood doctor to see the lad. This doctor diagnoses the case at once as appendicitis, and states that an operation within twenty-four hours is imperative. The young man is told that the operation will cost $200 and his hospital bill about $50. The young man has not the money and is a comparative stranger in the city. He explains his circumstances and symptoms fully to the visiting nurse. She doubts the necessity for an immediate operation and suggests that another doctor be called before an operation is decided on. The second doctor diagnoses the disease as quinsy, treats it accordingly, and the patient recovers without the $250 operation. Did the nurse do right? Is this a case where the nurse's loyalty to the doctor and loyalty to the patient's interests conflict?

14. A doctor calls a certain office asking for a visiting nurse to be sent to a patient suffering from gastric ulcer. He wishes the visiting nurse to administer a nutrient enema at stated intervals, to be preceded by a soap and water injection. After a few visits the nurse sends the following written report to the doctor:

"Dear Dr. X:—I have attended this afternoon Miss Y. She appears more bloodless than ever; her respiration resembles that of bad dropsy. The nutrient enema given this morning was rejected after three hours without appearance of slightest change, color, etc. Rectal tube used ten inches. No resistance to injection. I think there is a block of fæces in intestine high. Before it is too late will you let me make a suggestion? That she have on abdomen for three hours, occasionally, hot linseed with a little turpentine, and after two days take one ounce castor oil every third day, for twelve doses. She has painful spasm and hemorrhoids after soap injection. Is not her anæmia the outcome of constipation, doctor? She says for three years she has not used cathartic medicine. Please bear with me if I tell you that in the past I have by cathartics perforated an ulcer rather than allow death by stoppage, since healing can be found for moving ulcers. I think Miss Y. desires to see you in the morning. Will you tell her your wishes regarding poultice? I hope to visit in the afternoon."

Signed, Mary—Visiting Nurse.

Comment on this report, stating your reason for disapproving of it in any particular. What desirable qualities did the writer of this note appear to show or lack? Should the nurse herself or the training school be held responsible for such faults as you detect in this nurse, judging from the above report?

15. A visiting nurse is assigned to visit patients who are insured by a certain insurance company. She responds to a call sent by the insurance office. The doctor is with the patient when she arrives. He tells her she is not needed. She states that she is required to visit all patients, on instruction from the insurance company. The doctor says he cares nothing about insurance companies or their rules, and states that he will not have a trained nurse interfering with any of his cases. The nurse tries to reason with him; he gets angry and states that if she insists on interfering with his patients he will resign from the case. The patient seems to be very ill. What should the nurse do?

16. A visiting nurse is called to an old lady patient by

a neighbor. She finds that the old man and woman live alone; both are ill in bed with influenza, the old lady having some kidney complication besides. Both are over eighty years of age and are living on a little pension which barely suffices for their daily needs. The nurse takes the temperatures of both patients, gives the old lady a bath, and does not return. The old couple are entirely dependent in their illness on such attention as a kind neighbor with a baby and family of small children can give them. Did the nurse do her full duty in this case? If not, outline what you think her method of procedure should have been, if she wished to do her best for the welfare of the old couple.

17. Does this clause in a nurse's pledge apply to visiting nurses: "That whatsoever you shall see or hear of the lives of men and women, whether they be your patients or members of their households, you will keep unviolably secret, whether you are in other households or among your own friends?" Is it possible for visiting nurses to keep this pledge? To what extent is it permissible for visiting nurses to discuss the domestic affairs of their patients? What restrictions should be observed in discussing cases with members of the board of managers, some of whom may be women or men who are not averse to gossip? Have the poor the same rights to have the privacy of their homes respected as the middle class or rich? Give reasons for your answer.

18. A visiting nurse is engaged by a family to assist at a birth and to visit the patient afterward. The doctor's manner when she arrives shows very plainly that he does not wish the nurse to assist him in any way. She offers to prepare a disinfectant solution for his hands, asks whether he wishes anything sterilized, etc. He gruffly declines all such suggestions and does not even

wash his hands before making an examination to determine progress of labor. What should the nurse do in such a case during the labor? If a septic condition follows the birth in such a case, and the nurse knows the doctor is careless or incompetent, what are her duties in the matter?

19. A visiting nurse is employed by a committee of ladies for service in a town of 3500. Two graduate nurses whose homes are in or near the town are practising there and are busy, a considerable part of their work being maternity nursing. The committee of ladies have raised by means of various social affairs about $300, before the visiting nurse arrives. They are to pay her $65 a month, but she is supposed to earn most of it. The committee announces through the press that they are providing a nurse for the poor. They announce to the visiting nurse that they expect her to secure as much work as she possibly can from people who are able to pay, and that the continuance of her service there depends on how much she herself can earn toward her own salary. Through their clubs and churches and friends the committee advertises the benefits of their visiting nurse, and prospective mothers are urged to secure her for service at birth and for as many hours daily therafter as they need. The visiting work, through the advertising given and the activity of the committee, enjoys a "boom;" the work of the two private nurses dwindles. They go to the visiting nurse and complain that she is cutting rates, spending whole days at cases, and taking away their work. She explains that she has to do this work in order to keep her position, and that the committee fixes the rates. What should the visiting nurse do and what should the private nurses do under such circumstances?

ETHICS AND PRIVATE NURSING

20. A nurse is called to nurse an only child, a boy of eighteen, who has typhoid fever. An uncle of the boy is the doctor. The boy hates his uncle, who seems rather tactless and incompetent, but the boy's parents insist on having his uncle treat him, and seem to trust him implicitly. The boy has a highly nervous temperament. He confides to the nurse his hatred of his uncle and his distrust of his professional ability. The case is very long and tedious. The temperature refuses to remain normal, and the doctor insists that nothing but fluids shall be given till the temperature is normal ten days. The doctor will not listen to any suggestion from the nurse. The boy chafes against being starved, grows more and more depressed and melancholy, and frequently declares his intention of committing suicide. The nurse, believing that more liberal feeding would help to relax the tension and relieve the intense mental depression, resolves to make false entries of temperature on the chart, to lead the doctor to believe the temperature was normal when it was not, in the hope that he would allow the boy to have more food. The nurse's plans succeed. The boy improves quickly and markedly. The doctor and everyone is pleased, but the nurse suffers horribly from remorse because of her deception in the case. What should the nurse have done under such circumstances?

21. A private duty nurse thinks she should be called to any case needing a special nurse in the hospital from which she graduated if her name appears at the top of the list on call in the school registry. The principal of the school refuses to take nurses in rotation from the registry, and reserves the right to choose nurses according to her ideas as to temperamental or other fitness for such

cases. The private nurse secures several signatures from graduates of the same school to a protest against what is termed "unfair discrimination" in calling nurses for special duty, and sends the protest to the principal and to the training-school committee. The committee refuses to take action in the matter. The principal still asserts her right to choice of nurses and states that any nurse who has conducted herself while on special duty so as to give satisfaction, who has shown her loyalty to the hospital and set an example to pupil nurses as to what a graduate nurse's conduct should be, need not fear but that she will get her fair share of calls for special nursing. Which party is right in this situation?

22. A nurse is asked to accompany a nervous patient on a visit to her sister in a neighboring city. The patient likes to dine at hotels and restaurants, expects the nurse to accompany her, but does not offer to pay for the expense, and evidently expects the nurse to pay for her own dinners. What should the nurse do?

23. A nurse is called to care for two elderly ladies who are ill with bronchitis. The maid, the only other member of the household, develops grippe and goes to her sister's. Outline the nurse's duties under such circumstances.

24. A graduate learns that a member of her alumna association is in the habit of charging $5.00 for ordinary care to a body after death, in addition to the regular rate by the day or week. The nurse who makes the extra charge maintains that she is entitled to a special fee for services rendered to the body after death. The other nurse disagrees. What is her duty in regard to the discovery that the demanding of a special fee for services after death is being practised by a graduate of her own school?

25. A nurse is called to a case of ptomaine poisoning in a young man in the country some eight miles from the city where the nurse is located. The nurse goes in the morning. The patient dies about four in the afternoon. The nurse returns to the city that evening and charges the family $5.00 for the eight hours in which she was there and $5.00 for going to the country. Comment on this nurse's action and attitude toward human needs, and tell how such incidents are liable to affect the general reputation of trained nurses and the demand for their services?

26. A doctor asks a nurse who has just returned from a case of scarlet fever to assist him at an operation the following morning. He insists that there is no danger. The nurse fears she might carry infection. What should she do when the doctor says he will assume all responsibility?

27. A nurse is caring for her sister, a maternity patient, on a Dakota farm. A young man is very ill on a ranch about five miles distant. The nearest doctor is twelve miles away. The young man is unable to void urine, and the request is made for the nurse to catheterize him. What should the nurse do? What general rules should a nurse observe in regard to the catheterization of male patients?

28. A nurse is called to care for an alcoholic male patient in a hotel in a small town. The patient is vomiting incessantly, and the heart is in exceedingly bad condition. Should a nurse respond to such calls? If so, what general rules of conduct should she be careful to observe while in the hotel? Mention some general rules which nurses should commonly observe when nursing in hotels, whether the patient be male or female.

29. A nurse is asked to dress in uniform and assist in

collecting money for the support of nurses in a tag-day affair on a public street. Several young women who are not nurses are also to dress in nurse uniforms and have charge of collection boxes in public places. What attitude should a nurse take toward such a proposition?

30. Mention some good reasons why nurses should restrict the wearing of their uniform to the sick-room and its immediate vicinity. Is it desirable for nurses *in uniform* to visit drug stores and ice-cream parlors in the vicinity of the hospital and remain there with other patrons while they partake of ice cream and other refreshments? Give reasons for or against wearing the uniform in such places.

31. A nurse on an obstetrical case in a wealthy private home finds that the husband is very indifferent to wife and baby. The wife worries a good deal over his neglect. He is very profuse in his attentions to the nurse, insists on her always dining with him and prolongs the meal hours as long as possible. The nurse knows how the wife feels about matters and is perplexed to know how to manage the situation. What suggestions can you offer her?

32. A graduate nurse has been for several weeks in a suburban town nursing two children. When the children are convalescent the mother decides to go to the neighboring city to spend the day with a friend and attend a meeting or social affair in the evening. She leaves the nurse in entire charge of the home. As soon as the mother has gone, the nurse telephones to the city and invites two friends to spend the day with her. She bribes the little girl not to tell her mother. Comment on this nurse's actions in this case. Would they tend to increase the confidence and respect accorded to trained nurses in that town?

33. A young graduate, on special duty in a hospital in a small city, is invited by the husband of her patient to go for an automobile ride, and to bring with her a certain pupil nurse who had relieved the special nurse and of whom the patient was fond. The ride is arranged. The patient's husband is salesman for a brewing concern. He has a married man, a friend of his, in the car when they start for the drive. A long drive is taken in the country, and on their return the car is halted at a roadside hotel and the party of four go inside for refreshments. The hour is late. Several other "joy-riders" are in the place drinking, and drinks are ordered for the nurses by the men. They have never been in such a place before, and as they do not know exactly what to do or how to get away they accept the drinks. A friend of the president of the hospital board happens into the road house, recognizes the nurses drinking with the two married men, and reports the matter to the president of the board. The president blames the principal of the school for laxity of discipline in allowing her nurses to go about late at night with married men of loose character. The principal is so heartbroken over the scandal that she resigns her position. Who was to blame throughout this incident? Should the nurses have gone for the ride? Having done so, how could they have prevented the unpleasant consequences? What restrictions should be observed in accepting invitations of this sort?

34. A lady happened into a hospital which kept a registry for its graduates, asking for a nurse immediately for a seriously ill patient. There were no nurses available at this registry. The lady used the hospital telephone to call another registry which promised to send a nurse at once. The nurse failed to appear in two and a half hours, and an exasperated member of the family secured

a nurse from still another registry. The nurse secured had been on the case about an hour when the nurse who had first promised to come came driving up in a taxicab, at noon, and was told that she was not needed. She was very indignant and sent the bill for the taxicab, which amounted to $1.95, to the family. They refused to pay it. She then wrote a most indignant letter to the superintendent of the hospital from which the first telephone call had been sent, demanding that the hospital pay the bill for the taxicab.

Write comments on this situation telling who was at fault, whether the nurse should have called the taxicab in daylight without asking the family about it, and who should have paid the bill in this case.

35. A nurse is called to a case of typhoid fever, when the patient becomes delirious and a second nurse is needed. When convalescence begins, the family wish to retain the second nurse called because the patient prefers her. What should the first nurse and the second nurse do under such circumstances?

36. In a certain case, similar to the above, the family settled the above question by retaining the first nurse, though they much preferred the second. The day after the second nurse left the case, the nurse who remained in charge of the case received a call to another typhoid fever case which was just developing and would probably last six weeks, while the case she was with would be concluded in a week. She suddenly tells the family that she must leave at once and does so, leaving behind her a bundle of soiled clothing which she tells the family they are responsible for having laundered and for sending to her. Comment on the nurse's actions in this case, showing where her ethical lack was and how such conduct affects the reputation of other graduates.

37. A patient, an elderly man, dies. The body is to be shipped out of the city for burial. The only daughter of the deceased is to accompany the body, leaving the widow, an elderly woman, alone. The daughter asks the nurse to stay with her mother till she returns from the funeral. There is nothing for the nurse to do but ordinary household duties and to serve as companion for the old lady. Should the nurse stay?

38. A nurse is called to a case on which there is another nurse who is careless and does very poor work, is exceedingly disagreeable, and will accept no suggestion as to change in methods. The family are not exactly satisfied with the first nurse, but say nothing to her about her work and evidently intend to tolerate her where they cannot admire, respect, or love her. The whole situation is exceedingly distasteful to the second nurse in her dealings with the first nurse. The patient is very seriously ill. What should the second nurse do?

39. A well-to-do family (not rich) living in an apartment house had occasion to call a nurse for the mother of the lady of the house, an old lady in the eighties, who was slowly dying of some form of cancer—no external wounds. The man of the house was obliged to take business trips out of the city which often kept him away for weeks. He thought a trained nurse would be a pleasant companion for his wife. The nursing duties were light, but he did not care to have his wife left alone. No maid was kept. The nurse came, a stern, unbending creature who literally took possession of the sick-room and, from the moment she entered, gave the lady of the house to understand that she would tolerate no trespassing on her domain. Neither did she intend to offer to do anything outside the actual care of the patient. There was no rise of temperature in the patient, yet she religi-

ously took the temperature three times a day, kept detailed charts and, so far as technical work was concerned, she apparently left nothing undone and did much that was unnecessary.

The situation was painfully tense. The old lady grieved at the thought that her daughter, who knew how she liked things done, could do nothing for her, that she was not allowed to have her with her as she had been accustomed to. The daughter prepared more elaborate meals for herself and the nurse than she would have done when she was alone, washed the dishes and waited on the nurse instead of on her mother. The nurse rocked hours each day in a rocking chair, reading or doing embroidery, but not once did she suggest to the lady of the house that she stay an hour or two with the patient while she washed dishes or prepared a meal.

At the end of two weeks the husband returned, and finding that his wife was working harder than before the nurse came and the mother missed her daughter so sorely, dispensed with the nurse's services. A few days later they secured an untrained woman who fitted into the household as if she belonged there, assisted the daughter with the nursing and with any other duty that had to be done, and remained with the family till the patient died.

What were the chief reasons for the failure of the trained nurse in this case?

40. A nurse is called to an obstetrical patient on the second day after the birth of the child. The baby's eyes are infected. The patient, privately to the nurse, blames the doctor, whom she declares was in a great hurry and did not take proper care of her and the child at delivery.

The doctor privately tells the nurse that the husband is to blame, that he had previously had gonorrhea and thought himself cured. What should the nurse do when questioned by the patient as to how the infection occurred, and when the patient is telling all her friends that the doctor's neglect is the cause of the trouble?

41. A nurse has made an engagement to nurse a maternity patient due, probably, the first week in October, the engagement to last two weeks. The last week in September the nurse received a call to nurse a case of typhoid fever that will probably last from four to six weeks. The doctor who is to have charge of the obstetrical case is a stranger to her. The doctor who calls her for the fever case is one who frequently employs her. Is she justified in giving up the shorter case and taking the longer? What are the gains and losses to be weighed in coming to a decision?

42. A nurse is called to care for a little girl five years old in her home. The child has not been trained to obey. She objects to taking food. The doctor is most anxious to have the child gain in weight, and leaves a tonic to increase appetite. The child kicks and rebels against every dose of medicine. The mother does not interfere either to hinder or help. How should the nurse manage to get the medicine taken? What can she do to overcome the difficulties in regard to getting the child to take more food?

43. A nurse is employed for two months in a home in which a child has scarlet fever. The patient is practically convalescent after three weeks, but because there are five other children in the home the family feel they must somehow contrive to keep the nurse till the doctor pronounces all danger to the other children past. The man earns $200 a month and pays the nurse half of it, besides her board and laundry. No maid is kept. What are the nurse's duties under such circumstances?

44. What can a nurse do to make a protracted convalescence less tedious for a boy of five; a boy of ten, and a boy of fifteen years of age; also for girls of the same age?

45. To what extent is it wise for a nurse to discuss politics or religion with her patients?

46. A nurse is called to a patient who is suffering from a nervous collapse, following weeks of social dissipation in which dances, drinking, midnight suppers and late hours had been indulged in. The patient finally was unable to continue the strain longer and went to bed, ill and full of remorse over her dissipation. She feels that she can never be forgiven for some things which she did, and the question of forgiveness preys on her mind. She wants to talk with a minister. The family tell the nurse that she must guard against the patient "getting excited over religion" and that the subject of religion must not be mentioned. The doctor does not seem to understand how the patient's mental condition is hindering her recovery. The family so firmly believe that a minister would do the patient harm that they would not consider having one called. How should the nurse manage such a situation?

47. A doctor (married) who frequently employs a nurse for private duty is inclined to be familiar in his manner. He visits the patient, presumably, but spends twice as much time with the nurse as with the patient. The nurse is afraid the patients will think she is to blame for the doctor spending most of the time spent in the call with her. She does not wish to offend the doctor because he sends her many calls, but she is determined that her name shall not be connected with this doctor's as a topic for neighborhood gossip. How shall she manage this problem?

48. A nurse is nursing an old lady in a home and is asked to prescribe for a child who is taken ill in the night, presumably with diarrhea. The family owe the doctor and do not wish to add to his bill till they can pay part of it. What should the nurse do?

49. A graduate nurse, on special duty in a hospital with a very seriously ill patient, is relieved several hours every day by a pupil nurse. The pupil nurse discovers that the graduate is falsifying her records, is recording duties done before they are done, nutrient enemata given that have not been given, etc., and that her method is to write up the records once or twice a day just previous to the time the doctor makes his visits. The pupil nurse reports this condition to the head nurse in charge of the department. What is the duty of the head nurse and of the institution in regard to this matter?

50. A graduate nurse in a smaller city has a friend who is a druggist. He suggests to her that she might throw favors in his direction, that there are ways of increasing drug orders, and that she might use her influence with other nurses to patronize him. The nurse knows that he frequently substitutes inferior drugs for those ordered. He frequently sends her bottles of perfume, cold cream, etc. Should the nurse accept such articles? What should her attitude be regarding the friend's suggestions?

CHAPTER XXVI

Cooperation for Wider Service

During her final year of training a nurse will probably hear more or less about the duties which she owes to her alumna association and to other associations of nurses. It is hard to define such duties or to generalize about them, because the situations of nurses differ so greatly and nurses so often have to choose between apparently conflicting claims of duty on their time. The joining of an alumna association should be regarded in the light of a privilege. An active alumna association has much to offer the young graduate. Among its advantages may be mentioned the following:

It fosters the spirit of comradeship and good-will.

It promotes the work-together spirit, the spirit of cooperation for the good of all graduates of the school.

It furnishes a means by which a nurse may keep in touch with the developments and progress of her own school.

It should tend to foster a spirit of loyalty to the school and devotion to its best interests.

It gives a sense of strength and courage to a nurse who might otherwise feel herself to be an isolated unit, whose failures or successes as a nurse were of no special interest to anyone.

It furnishes an opportunity through which a nurse may assist her comrades as she could not assist as an isolated individual.

It frequently affords opportunities for a nurse to participate in programs and listen to lectures on newer methods or movements, thus stimulating in a nurse the desire to keep abreast with the times and to continue her studies.

It offers the natural opportunity for social activities, which most nurses need.

It enables a nurse to make her influence count where movements for social betterment are concerned.

Other advantages might be cited, but these indicate the possibilities of a well-managed alumna association. That all these advantages are not found in every alumna association is true. The association is just what the graduates make it. Not infrequently the older members are inclined to form in groups by themselves, and the same may be true of younger members. Where such conditions develop, the good influences which the association might exert are greatly lessened and its usefulness crippled.

In many smaller cities the county association of nurses serves many of the purposes of an alumna association, and affords a natural means of communication with nurses of various schools.

The objects of an association are always important. Many of these objects are planned chiefly with the idea of mutual benefit and improvement in mind. This idea to a certain extent should be present, but when an association exists solely for the benefit of itself and its members, its field of usefulness is limited and its influence comparatively slight. Too radical effort on the part of one set of nurses to improve another set may easily defeat its object, and material benefits are often hard to show. Where, however, an association demonstrates that it is working not solely for the benefit of its members, but for the utmost service it can render to humanity, it furnishes a stronger appeal to individual members than any mutual benefit plan can supply.

"To promote, by cooperation, the effectiveness of the nursing profession and through it the good of the community" is the object of an association of English nurses that has rendered conspicuous service in a variety of ways. This tersely stated object is well worthy of consideration. It embodies much.

One or two illustrations out of hundreds that might be mentioned are cited to show how far-reaching are the benefits that a local association of nurses may render. In a certain small city of about 40,000 a local association, because of the vision of one of its members, became convinced that a dispensary was needed to which poorer patients could come for free examination and treatment. Their first appeal was to the doctors of the community. The appeal was backed up by numerous descriptions of patients, of whom the nurses knew, who should be helped by dispensary treatment. The doctors agreed to cooperate and to contribute their services. Next they appealed to the hospital for a room and for other assistance. The hospital could not immediately offer accommodations for the dispensary, but promised to when the opening of its new nurse's home would make it possible. It offered to assist by sending one or two senior nurses during dispensary hours, and in other ways as might be necessary. Nothing daunted, the nurses set about to find a room which could be rented. The room was found in the basement of a store. They raised, by subscription among themselves, the doctors and interested citizens, a couple of hundred dollars for a modest equipment. Finally they hunted up many of the patients and brought them personally to the dispensary. The hospital has since taken over the dispensary, and its value to the community has been unquestioned. One of its indirect results was to increase profoundly the respect and admiration for trained nurses in that community. The object of working for the good of the community does much to maintain that wholesome interest that is essential for the highest success.

In another smaller city, the county association of nurses subscribed and collected funds to put a visiting nurse at work for the summer months. The need was so thoroughly demonstrated that an organization of citizens was easily effected to continue the work.

Ye Have Need of Patience.—It is a common failing of nurses as of many other workers, that they clamor for immediate benefits or results from some organization with which they have allied themselves. If these benefits are not speedily forthcoming they lose interest. Many of the results which accrue from such organizations are indirect, and a nurse very often benefits in proportion to the amount of herself that she puts into it. The enriching of one's own life, the finding of a channel through which our best desires may find expression, is a benefit to every nurse who honestly wants to make the world a better place to live in.

"Learn to labor and to wait" is an admonition frequently needed in this age when the tendency in many places is to expect to reap a harvest before a seed has had time to germinate and really take root.

The spirit of intolerance with those whose opinions differ from ours is frequently seen in nurses' associations, and it is a spirit which every nurse who really desires the best things for an association should try to suppress. There are truths in the following quotation from a popular weekly paper which are worthy of earnest consideration, lest we become "self-opinionated," censorious, and uncharitable in our judgments of the motives of other workers who have every right to an opinion of their own.

"We are sometimes tempted into thinking that this would be a very much better and happier world if other folks would only agree with us and see things as we do. But really the chances are that this tremendously radical change in affairs would be no improvement. This conflict of judgment and clash of opinions is not the bad thing that we sometimes take it to be. It is a way—yes, even a divine way, of progress. The radical who stirs up our inert conservatism may not be altogether agreeable to us, but we may need him just the same, and the man who opposes some of our pet plans and policies may be our good, though much disguised, friend. To agree to differ is sometimes much better than to agree. Conflicts of judgment will never cease, but contempt of other folks' judgment ought to. 'You are entitled to a point of view,' said a lecturer, 'but not to announce it as the center of the universe.'"

The peril of narrowness has been mentioned before. It is one which threatens every nurse and is one which membership in a nurses' association should help to combat. It should help to give her a view of national movements, and an opportunity to cooperate in many of the broader programs and efforts for human betterment. There is, however, a real danger of a nurse joining so many nursing associations that she does not count for much in any of them. Her energies are so dissipated, spread out so thinly, that she fails to accomplish anything of real value in any of them. There is also the danger of becoming so engrossed in nursing affairs that one has neither time nor energy left to give to any other good movements. Nurses who commit the blunder of mingling with nurses and of thinking of nursing exclusively or to the neglect of other friends or causes, cannot fail to grow narrow in their views, and this is reflected in their conversation. They "talk shop" constantly because they know of little else besides nursing to talk about.

If for no other reason than for her salvation from petty prejudices, selfishness and narrowness, every nurse needs to connect herself with some cause, some interest that is not connected with nursing. To the man or woman who has allowed himself (or herself) to become engrossed with *one* interest, or has allowed *one* cause to loom up and fill the whole horizon, there is a constant temptation to go to harmful extremes, and to regard those who have more varied interests in life, and a different viewpoint, as enemies to the cause they have at heart.

A variety of interests in life helps one greatly to form a just estimate of relations and proportions and values, and very often shows that the thing we have been urged to throw our whole energies into has not in itself the possibilities of enough returns in good to ourselves, our associates or the commonwealth, to justify spending much time or effort on it.

Beyond all this there is found in the person who has read widely and is well informed on a variety of lines of activity, the person who is "broad" in his viewpoint of life as a whole, a geniality, generosity, a freedom from petty prejudice and suspicion, that gives to him a genuine charm of character, much to be coveted. In this breadth of interest there is also a veritable bulwark against loving one's own way too well, and the temptation to go to extremes on any question.

There are, perhaps, no reminders which nurses as a body need more frequently than that they should try to see both sides of a question before coming to conclusions; that they should avoid rushing to extremes; that they should study to keep always an open mind, and avoid letting petty prejudices possess them.

If one is to successfully accomplish this, one must have one or more interests outside of the nursing world and cultivate acquaintance with "many men of many minds."

No nurse is doing justice to herself who does not ally herself with some other great movement, social or religious, to help her to keep a proper balance in her life, to help her to see nursing in its true proportions and in its true relation to other great uplift movements.

Conferences and meetings with social service and charity workers are always broadening and educative. There are many points at which the work of the nurse and other social service workers touch, and it is important that a nurse be able to appreciate the work and the viewpoint of social workers who are making large contributions to state and community betterment.

Women's clubs in many cities are doing a work that is far-reaching and valuable. They are influencing public sentiment and legislation in a variety of ways. An active club devoted to earnest work is a good thing for any nurse to belong to, who has time to give to it. The women in such clubs represent to a large degree the great field which private nurses serve, and it is well worth while to get their viewpoint regarding nursing problems. Incidentally the nurse who is a member of such a club has frequent opportunities to give the "lay members" her viewpoint and to secure their cooperation in improving conditions, where nurses alone would be powerless to effect such improvement.

Working with Men.—Whatever other organizations a nurse belongs to, she should endeavor to become a member of at least one organization in which men and women are working together toward a common end. The masculine viewpoint on many problems is well worth having; in many circumstances it is essential to a well-balanced judgment. Better social and community conditions are only secured as men and women work together. The millennium will not be ushered in by women alone, or by men alone, but by men and women working together and working with God.

Suggested Subject for Written Work.—At a public meeting held to discuss the passage of a law restricting the use of habit-forming drugs, the promoters of the bill presented a strong letter from a graduate nurse. The letter especially called attention to the use of habit-forming drugs among nurses and hospital internes. It stated that not only were nurses addicted to habit-forming drugs themselves, but that they often procured them for patients who craved them. Also that they gave drugs to patients under their care and without authority, in order to obtain restful nights, and that in many cases the patient's recovery was seriously retarded thereby.

What should be the attitude of the alumna association toward a nurse who is a member of the association and who makes public statements of this kind? Has an alumna association any responsibility in regard to investigating or disproving such statements?

QUESTIONS FOR DISCUSSION OR REVIEW

1. How much should a member of an alumna association be expected to do in the association beyond paying her dues and attending such meetings as she conveniently can?

2. Mention some obstacles commonly encountered in carrying on alumna association work?

3. If a few older members of a county association dominate everything, and use up the time for discussion at every meeting, what is the duty of younger graduates in regard to such an association?

4. If the members of one alumna association assume airs of superiority over graduates of other schools, in a county organization, and constantly insinuate that the training given in other schools in the same county is inferior, what is the duty of a graduate of one of the so-called inferior schools to the association, three out of five officers being of the "snobbish" or "superior" school?

5. What is the cause of "cliques" or factions in nurse's organizations? In what ways are they a detriment and how can they be prevented or eliminated?

6. How would you answer this request? "I would like to have some suggestion as to how to keep up interest in an alumna association and its meetings."

"Our association has been organized almost two years, we have twenty-four members; sometimes we have a quorum, sometimes we do not; and seldom more than enough to hold a meeting. I have recently been elected president and am anxious to build it up."

7. If a nurse who is a stranger in a city attends a few meetings of a county association and finds the time occupied with trivial details and the meetings most uninteresting, her opinion neither asked for nor apparently desired on any question, what is her duty in regard to such an association? Is she justified in considering attendance at such meetings a waste of time which she otherwise might profitably employ, and in

ceasing to attend? Should she be censured for not attending under such circumstances?

8. A nurse of rather indolent habits was accustomed to refuse to do various duties, such as keeping the patient's room neat, carrying the tray from kitchen to the invalid's room and back, filling the hot-water bottles for patients, etc., and always gave as her reason "the registry doesn't allow us to do such things." Finally she refused on one occasion to get up at night to give a drink to a child patient who was inconsiderate enough to become thirsty at night, and the child's aunt got up and got the drink. The aunt reported the matter to the registry, mentioning the various things which the nurse had said the registry didn't allow nurses to do. The registrar stated that no such rules existed in regard to the duties mentioned. The registry was controlled by the graduates of the school. What attitude should an alumna association assume under such circumstances?

9. It becomes known to members of an alumna association that one of their members is addicted to the use of morphine. She is practically under the influence of the drug all the time, yet is doing private nursing. Has the alumna association any responsibility in regard to this matter. What is their duty in regard to the nurse herself, to the public, and to the association? How should such a matter be handled?

10. Of what ethical failure is a nurse guilty who in a letter to a newspaper makes serious charges in regard to an organization, institution, or individual and refuses to sign her name to the letter? Should any individual make serious statements for public reading or discussion who is not willing to back up such statements with his name?

Lord, fill our minds to the brim with truth and love. From our hearts root out all vanity, pride, prejudice, and bitterness. Keep us from feeling that other people ought to be just like us. Make us large-minded, like thyself, taking pleasure in the beautiful varieties of life, and appreciative of diverse human values. Remove from us all bigotry, uncharity, harshness, and the unconscious hypocrisy of self-will and secret laudation. Relax the false strain that converts our tongues into threshing-flails, and keeps our souls seething and boiling with blame and faultfinding. Make us glad that God reigns, even when we do not. Make us a little shy of our own wisdom and always hospitable to other people's suggestions. Show us the hidden sore of sin deep in our own hearts, and cure that first of all.

—From a Veteran Pastor's Prayers.

INDEX

Featured Titles from Westphalia Press

Made in the USA
Monee, IL
04 November 2026

67383078R10184